DIGNITY & DEMENTIA: CARPE DIEM

My journals of living with dementia

MARY BETH WIGHTON

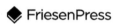 FriesenPress

Suite 300 - 990 Fort St
Victoria, BC, V8V 3K2
Canada

www.friesenpress.com

ISBN
978-1-5255-7089-6 (Hardcover)
978-1-5255-7090-2 (Paperback)
978-1-5255-7091-9 (eBook)

1. HEALTH & FITNESS, DISEASES, ALZHEIMER'S & DEMENTIA

Distributed to the trade by The Ingram Book Company

My Dawnie Girl – this book is dedicated to you.
From the deepest of my heart I thank you for
embracing our life with carpe diem.

"The most important thing is, even when we're apart …
I'll always be with you … "
Winnie the Pooh

My sister once told that I would meet some extraordinarily special people along this journey. How true she was. Jessica Luh Kim- You changed the course of my life. Thank you for your endless support and teaching me the fact that I am the expert. Lisa Poole –You are a constant reminder of the necessity for tenacity to affect change. It truly is an honour to call you my friend. And to the countless other special people who have helped me to live carpe diem-thank you.

CONTENTS

YEAR ONE

I Have What?

Date: September 5th, 2012, 9:00 a.m.
St. Mary's Hospital, Kitchener, Ontario, Canada

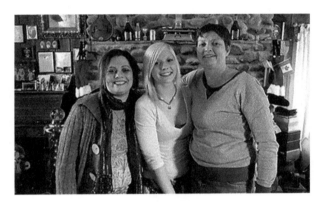

Dawn, Brianna, Me

As I drove us to the 9:00 a.m. meeting with the Geriatrician, many thoughts ran through my head. Here we go, another appointment with another doctor. One more stupid test. I hate when they ask me to write down the clock time because I know what time it is. I'm looking forward to my Timmy's coffee.

Once Dawn and I arrived at the hospital, we grabbed a coffee and headed off to the waiting room of the Geriatrician area. I asked myself, "How can I only be 45 years old and be sitting here?" Within minutes we were led into the examination room and the nurse arrived. Same old, same old. It really bothered me that after years of battling serious

1

depression, memory loss and behavioural changes, no one has provided me with a sound medical diagnosis. That was all about to change.

Nurse Julie began the mini–mental state examination (MMSE). Sure enough, there were the questions about time. I uttered to her that I don't have a problem with time. We continued. Finally, the last of 30 questions lay in front of me. My mind was tired, and it had become hard to stay focused. I didn't have the brain power to answer any more questions – we were finished. After asking Dawn and I a few more questions about my health, she disappeared to tally the results.

Soon, the door opened, and Nurse Julie appeared with the doctor. Everyone sat down. The doctor immediately started to discuss the results of the MMSE. Six months ago, I had taken the same test and scored 24. Today, my score was 18 – an obvious, significant decrease.

I'm not sure of all the things she discussed, but I do remember this: *"You have Frontotemporal Lobe Dementia or FTD."* Whoa.... no one has ever used those words before. I knew I was cognitively impaired but what was this FTD thing? The doctor went on to explain more about FTD including that my amount of education will help. More blurred talk. FTD is a rare form of dementia and is incurable.

Dawn and I looked at each other. Could this really be happening? More blurred talk. You will not be able to drive any more effective immediately. What? O.K. This is now serious. More blurred talk.

I stopped hearing the rest of the conversation. The only thing I could hear in my head was, *"You can't drive."* You don't have a driver's license!" I started to see red. I flew out of my chair and threw some papers in the garbage. I stormed out of the office trying me best to slam the door shut. I tried a few times.

I continued to the hospital hall and stopped. I began to pace up and down mumbling to myself. How could this be? How can I have dementia? How can my license be removed? How can my license be removed? How can I have dementia? My head was in a swirl. I continued to pace.

My cell phone rang, and it was Dawn asking where I was, if I was o.k. And for me to come back into the room. No! I'm not coming back into the room because I don't want to hear anymore. I continued to pace.

Eventually, Dawn came out of the examination room and approached me in the hall. We said nothing and I handed my car keys to her. We headed out towards the car. Dawn proceeded to take my usual seat at the wheel, and I took her usual seat as a passenger. FTD had changed our lives forever.

The Importance of Tradition

Date: December 14th, 2014

I love tradition. I come from and am part of a family of traditions. Growing up, holidays were always a time of making the same yummy recipes, putting up the same Christmas tree, visiting the same people, telling the same funny stories, and putting up the same homemade Christmas stockings for Santa to fill.

As I grew older, I took with me many of these traditions and eventually introduced them to my own family. One of my favorite tradition is decorating our Christmas tree. Eight years ago, when we celebrated our first family Christmas together, we began the tradition of going to a local tree farm to buy our Christmas tree.

Now remember, global warming had not affected the weather as much, so we had something called "snow." The tradition began at the house with the pulling on of big coats, boots, hats, mitts, and snow pants. You always hoped you didn't have to go to the washroom! Our two dogs, Leo and Riley also had a special outfit for the event. Both dogs had their sweaters and Christmas bells put on them. We laughed as they began their dance trying to get the bells off their legs.

We all piled into the van and the Christmas singsong began. The tree farm was close so in no time we arrived at a busy scene. People, trees, dogs, and snow. What a wonderful, chaotic place! We quickly filed out of the van and rushed to the opening of the farm.

This is where I would put Brianna into the sleigh we had brought and began to "mush." With the dogs prancing beside us, we began to inspect the many trees until finding the perfect one. At a young age,

I always encouraged Brianna to be independent. With my assistance, she would lay down on the cold snow and begin to saw the tree trunk. Down it would come with a collective "yeahhhh" from all of us.

We always liked to count the rings on the tree to know how old it was. For some reason, this was important. The tree would then be moved onto the sled to be towed back to the point of entry so we could pay for it. I always loved that walk back. The cold, the snow falling softly, the sounds of the dog's bells, and the excited chatter of my family. I felt at peace.

Once we arrived back, we would proceed into the small building to have hot apple cider. How wonderful it tasted. Brianna would then walk through the aisles of Christmas decorations and pick out the one she would like to take home with her. Every year, Brianna still picks out one Christmas ornament to adorn the tree. The tree would then be strapped to the roof of the van, and we would all pile back into it and head for home. From the roof, it would be moved into the garage for a day, so it had time to fall.

Once it is time to decorate the tree, family members take on specific roles. Dawn is the individual who hands out the tree ornaments to Brianna. She also has the especially important job of ensuring the tree is straight and if not, to coordinate the efforts to make it so. For some reason, our tree always seems to have a bit of a tilt. Brianna is the "hanger." It is her role to take the ornaments from Dawn and then find a special place on the tree for each and everyone. Dawn usually helps with instructions from the couch.

My role starts at the very beginning and goes to the end of the process. It begins by taking out all the boxes from storage and moving them into the family room. Then, from the garage, I take the Christmas tree into the house and put it into the tree stand. Next, I put a string of lights around the tree and make sure it looks even. Then my girls join me, and the decorating begins.

During the time in my life when I travelled around the world for work, I collected Christmas ornaments. Over the years, I have accumulated some beautiful and unique ornaments. Our family tradition is for me to is take each of these ornaments, prior to their positioning on the tree, and to provide the history of the ornament. It comes with the where and when I obtained these special treasures. Each year, bulbs from South Africa, Mexico, England, The Netherlands, Ireland, Texas, and Bethlehem are dusted off and placed in their spot of honour.

The other special bag that is brought out from its box is that containing Brianna's homemade ornaments. We all laugh and smile as we pick up each ornament and Dawn reminisces of the stories behind the little gems.

The final, most important moment is shared with Brianna and me. It is the adorning of the tree with the Christmas angel. When Brianna was little, I used to lift her up and she would place it on the top of the tree. But, now that she is 18, I just stand beside her as she does her work. And of course, a picture is taken of the yearly event.

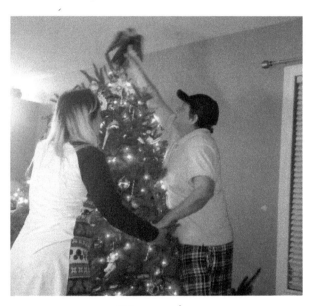

Brianna and me

Today, the three of us enjoyed this special day of Christmas tree decorating. Unfortunately, for the last three years we no longer venture to the tree farm but rather buy a cut tree from a lot.

Today's event was a bit different as we added a new element to it. For the first time, we videotaped it. Without saying it, we sensed the importance of capturing this beautiful moment this year. We are keenly aware that we do not know what FTD will bring over the next year. In fact, this year, a few variations had to take place to work around FTD. Brianna took over my role of ensuring that the tree was straight and properly secured. My sense of frustration was high, and I found it hard to tighten the tree holder bolts. Also, there were fewer decorations on the tree this year. It is so easy to be over stimulated that less is always better - even on the Christmas tree.

I must say a bit of a sense of relief has come to me. No matter what life brings to me, I know stories of the Christmas ornaments will be passed down through generations. The important tradition of the tree decorating will continue - no matter what.

Accepting My Diagnosis

December 17, 2012

If you believe 2012 doomsday theorists, the earth as we know it will end in 4 days on December 21, 2012. Whether it is from the end of the Mayan calendar or some incredible planetary collision, life on earth will end. Television movies depicting the end play repeatedly. The news captures religious fanatics holding their signs high to "repent." It has made me pause and wonder.

I do not believe in 2012 doomsday. I believe God has his own agenda.

It is in such stark comparison I contemplate my own inevitable death. Upon my diagnosis of FTD, I immediately went to my computer and began to research this foreign word. As I read through the text of symptoms, I eventually hit the words "Inevitably FTD will culminate in profound disability and death."

The average life expectancy is anywhere from 2-10 years with the mean of 8. I reread this line of text numerous times. Three months since my diagnosis, these words continue to sink in.

I've known for years, there was something seriously wrong with me. I just didn't know what it was. Finally, I had a diagnosis to this terrible thing. My emotions have ranged from disbelief to anger to sadness.

The one thing that has remained constant from the start is my desire to live life to its fullest and with dignity. At the bottom of my calendar page, I have written the well-known line, "Live each day as if it's your last." But, what does that really mean?

Words are just that – words. It is how we live those words that really matters.

Each day, I wake up and count my blessings and thank God. I try to be gentler with my words; tell my loved ones I love them; help as much as I can; and not hesitate to take up people's invitations to an adventure. I ask myself, am I correctly prioritizing things I must complete? I have begun to reach out to some dear old friends who I have lost contact with. I have told special people in my life that they are special, and my life is richer because they are in it. I do not take these relationships for granted. Laughter has become more important to me and I look to find and share things that will earn a smile. I continue to work hard to ensure that my family is left in the best circumstances it can be. I reach out to organizations that can help me move through challenges. And ultimately, each day, I try to give as much as I can to help in the fight against dementia.

I ponder about what my purpose of life is. Is helping in this fight it? Regardless, I will continue to live each day the best I can. I have accepted my diagnosis. It is the helping of others to aid in their acceptance of my diagnosis that is paramount.

My great niece, Teighan, recently presented me with a beautiful painting she had done herself. On it, she painted the words, "Carpe Diem." I have hung her painting up near the entrance of our home. As each person enters, I wish for them to join me in seizing the day and place no trust in tomorrow.

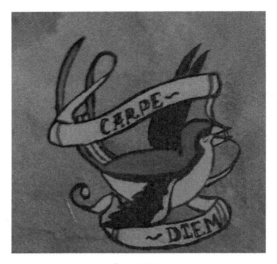

Carpe Diem

My Wednesday Morning Friend

Date: October 25th, 2012

The doorbell rang cutting the silence of the house. As I opened the door, a tall grey-haired woman filled the door frame. Immediately, I was drawn in by her warm eyes and her smile. I knew I would like her.

One week prior, Dawn had posted a classified on the KIJI website:

"We are a female couple in the Kitchener area. My partner has been diagnosed with Dementia- she is in her mid-40's. I am seeking a volunteer who can come into our home for 2-3 hours, play cards with my spouse, chit chat, have coffee, maybe go for lunch (we would treat) and share some laughs. I work from home, so I am here as well in my office. If you are interested, please contact the writer. Must have a criminal reference check."

I opened the door, and let her in. I introduced myself and she told me her name was Sharyn. We proceeded to the kitchen table where the interview would take place. The intent of today's meeting was to talk with each other and decide if we saw ourselves as a match. I had not interviewed someone in a few years, so I was a bit nervous. Over a cup of coffee, we proceeded to tell each other about ourselves. As we did so, the other person would ask questions, pulling more specific information out.

Sharyn's story was simple. She wished to volunteer her time. Sharyn told me she was a 66 years old retired nurse and a grandmother. She eagerly shared with me stories about her grand-babies and of her former days working in the hospital. I could tell she was a lover of people. Unbeknownst to Sharyn, I was more interested in the energy she projected than what she used to do for a living. And I liked the raw, positive energy she gave off.

Sharyn asked specific questions about FTD and the medication I was taking to help stave off its symptoms. A few times, she mentioned my young age of 46 years. She would gently shake her head.

After about 1.5 hours, we begin to wind down the meeting. It ended with a blunt question from her to me: *"Well, if you like me and want me, I can come next week."* And in that moment our relationship began.

Since that time, Sharyn has come every Wednesday at 10:30. She usually stays 2 to 2.5 hours. During this time, we converse on topics which range the gamut. I have learned about her growing up in Kitchener, having her children, and spending time with her grand babies. She discusses her relationships with her siblings and latest bowling score. She is a busy lady.

In return, I pull out my ancestry books, and tell her of the Wighton's' coming from Scotland generations ago. Stories of being the baby of a family of 8 children come tumbling out of my mouth. Imagine raising all those children! We laugh. I confide in her the plight of my Mom, who has Alzheimer's. And of my father who is her 85-year-old caregiver. Both of whom moved into a retirement home within the last month.

The first game we played was Scrabble. But, with our chit-chatting, it was hard to follow the game. The next week, I introduced her to the board game Sequence. She loved it! And we were hooked. Discussion on how much her granddaughter would like the game ensued.

Last week, December 12th, as Sharyn was starting to leave, Dawn asked her to wait a moment. From the kitchen, she came towards

Sharyn with a Christmas tin. Oh boy, Sharyn is one lucky girl. In the tin held a dizzying array of yummy homemade Christmas treats. The Christmas tin was a small token of appreciation.

Sharyn fills the Wednesday morning silence with laughter and warmth. My world is a better place because of her.

The Lucky Ticket – Not!

Date: December 20th 2012

I'm not much of a gambler. Once in a blue-moon, I like to buy a lottery ticket. I carefully choose my numbers, cross my fingers, and hope for the best. Then I play the fun game of "If I won a million dollars I would ...." Unfortunately, I never seem to pick the right numbers.

This also seems to be the case for when I made a gamble on what life insurance coverage I should choose. Back in 2005, things were busy in our lives. We had recently become partners in a business, Brianna had started grade six, and we were doing the normal things parents usually do.

Being critical ill was far from our minds.

I was in good shape - 5 ft 8 inches, 141 lbs., and a non-smoker. My only medical history of concern was heart disease. My Dad had two triple-bypasses by the time he was 75. Other than that, we Wighton's are a fine species.

Still, we felt it prudent to get some coverage "just in case." We met with an insurance agent from a well-known insurance company and he went through the packages we could invest in.

Critical illness insurance was founded in 1983 in South Africa under the name dread disease insurance. Typical critical illness insurance products refer to policies where the insurer pays the policyholder a pre-determined lump sum cash payment if the policyholder is diagnosed with a critical illness listed in the policy.

What is interesting is that the actual conditions covered depend on the market need for cover and competition amongst insurers. This determines the "norm." To put it another way, the diseases that most people are likely to get are put on the list and prioritized.

For us, it boiled down to two polices: 1) basic critical illness insurance and 2) critical illness insurance. This is kind of like when someone hands you two scratch tickets and asks you which one you want. You make your pick and scratch it off to see if you are a winner. I chose ticket number one – basic critical illness insurance. I chose the wrong ticket.

My insurance policy coverage only includes the following: 1) cancer 2) coronary artery bypass surgery 3) heart attack and 4) stroke. Remember, this list is based on what most people are like to get. Who would have thought at the age of 45 I would pull the unlucky ticket of Frontotemporal Lobe dementia (FTD)? But I did.

When I was first diagnosed, I thought to myself – its o.k. I have critical illness and life insurance. Of course, I didn't remember my coverage would not do that – cover me, because I did not have one of the four diseases listed within the policy. When I retrieved my paperwork out of our lock box, I quickly began to read it. It then hit me – hard – I had picked the wrong ticket. I was horrified.

It is one thing to place a $5 bet on a lottery ticket and loose. It's another thing to pay a monthly premium and lose. The second coverage plan I did not choose had dementia on the list for a payout disease. For a few dollars more each month, I could have had this policy and coverage. Hindsight being 20/20, I wish I had chosen the other policy product.

I started to cry. How can this be happening? I have just been diagnosed with dementia and I do not have critical life insurance that covers it. I flew into a rage. Dawn went for cover as I began to throw things around. I just could not handle it. I felt like I had failed my family. I hung my head down in shame.

Dawn and I are like so many other couples our age. We have a mortgage, car payments, a child at home, and are doing our best with balancing today and tomorrow's financial needs. From what we understand about the disease, Dawn will eventually become my primary care giver. How will she do that, work, and do everything else? And how about just spending time with me while the disease has not ravaged my body and mind.

So now what? Dawn and I will continue to do our best each day. Just like we always do. Dawn goes off to work each day; we continue to receive bills; and we continue to pay them.

However, it is with a heavy heart that she sits at her desk. Her work calls are interrupted by her own thoughts of wondering how I am, what I am doing, and if I am all right. She is not at that desk because she wants to be but out of necessity.

How different our lives would be if dementia had been on the basic coverage and we had received a large lump of cash. According to Alzheimer Society Canada, in 2011, 747,000 of Canadians 65 or older were living with cognitive impairment, which includes dementia. What is terrifying is that by 2031, this figure will increase to 1.4 million.

So, the obvious question is when does dementia get put on the basic coverage list?

If I did win a million dollars by picking the right numbers, I know exactly what I would do. I would have Dawn retire from her job and I would take her and Brianna to exotic, fascinating places in the world.

But more importantly, I would have her right beside me each day enjoying the simple pleasures of life. Because that is the real winning scenario. Enjoying time with the one you love without any financial concerns.

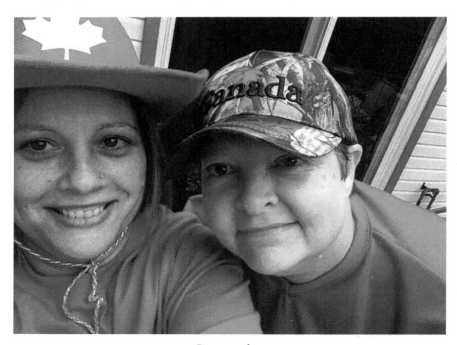

Dawn and me

Big Sister

Date: December 12th 2012

sis·ter (s s t r)

n.

1. A female having the same parents as another or one parent in common with another.

Well, that's one way to define sister. But that is not how I would define my sister Debbie. There is so much more to "sister" than biological ties.

My parents had three boys, then Debbie, then three more boys, then me. Debbie and I were obviously the minority of the family. When I was born, I would imagine Debbie being thankful to finally have another female amongst all those boys.

My memories of her start at a young age. Things were different back in the old days. Kids would share not only bedrooms but beds. Debbie and I shared a bed. There are 13 years between us. So, she was already a teenager when I arrived. I did not wet my bed for long, but I do remember it happening once, and my dear sister getting me up, cleaning me and changing our bed sheets. Never a crossword did she utter.

Another time, I was extremely sick and in bed. I began to cry and yell for help as I started to vomit in the bed. One of my brothers was on the telephone outside the door. He did not move to help me. It was my Debbie who came running in to save the day. Each time she came in and out of the bedroom, she chastised the brother who was on the telephone. But for me, I only received gentle words as she cleaned me up and tucked me back into bed.

As we grew older, Debbie began to date Ron, now her husband. She continued to have her eye on me. One birthday, Ron banged on the door. He was here to take Debbie and I apple picking. Every September, I still think of that wonderful day.

Debbie soon married and began to have children of her own. All the while she would take advantage of opportunities to help educate me on life, its challenges, and possible solutions.

13

Our Mom found it difficult to discuss things every woman should know. Debbie would check-in with me ensuring I understood the milestones of change.

Eventually, I caught up with her and reached adulthood. Certainly, a confusing and exciting time. My big sister shared with me her philosophy on leading a good life and the importance of God. Her good actions challenged me to think about my own actions which were not always so good. She did not have words chastising me but rather words to encourage me. It is hard to believe, but I do not remember ever a time when we spoke crossly to each other. Imagine!

In the last few years, dark days entered my life. Through it all, Debbie continued to reach out to me, encouraging me and showing her love for me. I deeply appreciated it.

Just this September, the time I always think about apple-picking with her and Ron, I was diagnosed with FTD. Debbie was one of the first people to call me up. I don't remember too much about what we talked about, but just that we cried together.

Just a few days after that telephone call, I received a package in the mail. It was from my big sister. In it was a treasure – her own, well-used and loved bible. Debbie was giving me something that she cherished deeply. I was humbled by her actions.

I am blessed to have such a sister. Debbie continues to reach out to her little sister, to help her during the journey she finds herself in.

Thank you, Debbie, – I love you.

- Your little sister.

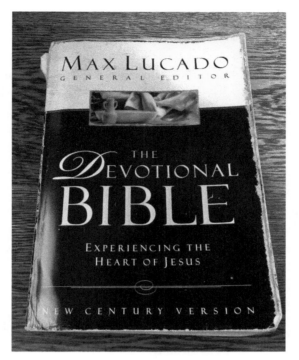

The Bible

Unconditional Love

Date: December 27th 2012

It all started on a cold, snowy, blistery night. It was our first real winter storm. We were all tucked in our home – Dawn was in bed asleep; Brianna was in her bedroom talking on the telephone and laughing.

That is what every 18-year-old should be doing. But Brianna was having a restless night and was finding it difficult to fall asleep. I too was longing for slumber which just didn't seem to come.

I was in my usual spot – on the couch with my dog Shiloh beside me. I was watching TV. I had been experiencing swallowing problems for most of the day. My saliva would collect in my mouth and some-what consciously my tongue would push the saliva down my throat.

The sides of my tongue were becoming raw as I continually rubbed it against my teeth to push the collection in my mouth down.

Dawn brought to me my mouthguard that I wear at night because I grind my teeth. It seemed to help somewhat, but irritated, I would pull it out for a while and then put it back in. This went on for hours.

During this time, I became aware of Brianna laughing. It was 1:30 in the morning and something in my brain told me to go upstairs and tell Brianna it was late, and she should say good night to her friend. When I opened her bedroom door, she looked up at me with surprise. In a stern voice I told her to hang up as it was late. Brianna complied.

I went back downstairs to continue being restless. It was about an hour later and I became thirsty. This swallowing thing was really getting to me and I went upstairs to get a glass of water. I saw Brianna's bedroom light on. I thought to myself, I told her to get to bed, why is she not doing it! So, I went in again. Brianna was quietly talking on the telephone. Again, she looked up at me in surprise.

It is at that moment, that I do not know what happened to me. I became my own worst nightmare. I began to yell at Brianna, telling her to get off the phone. She told me she couldn't sleep, and she wasn't loud or hurting anyone. That was not the answer I wanted to hear. I became enraged. How dare her! I saw red. I do not know what I said to Brianna. I do know my words were very hurtful and very disrespectful. And the words just kept coming from my mouth and coming and coming.

Dawn awoke from her slumber and ran to the bedroom to see what was going on. My rage continued towards Dawn. Once again, I do not know what I said, just that I was mean.

Dawn tried to talk with me in a reasonable way. She informed me Brianna was having trouble sleeping and had been in to see her three times that evening. I didn't care. I just wanted to keep yelling. I moved back downstairs to my couch. My girls followed me. We were all now upset and began to yell at each other. Words from my mouth just kept coming. I was mean. I was terribly mean.

I needed to leave – to get out of the house as quickly as I could. It was now 2:30 in the morning and the snow was coming down heavily.

I began to put my boots and coat on. Dawn tried to get in front of the door to stop me. I screamed at her to get out of my way and let me out.

Somehow, I managed to get by her and began to head off into the night wearing my pajamas, a coat and my boots. There was no stopping me. I didn't look back. Into the dark I went.

I'm not sure when it happened, but I began to sob uncontrollably. It came to me that I wanted to get out of the house because I needed to stop hurting my family. I kept walking. I did not have a goal in mind, I just knew I had to keep walking.

Between sobs, I began to mumble to myself – it truly has "started." Frontotemporal Lobe Dementia (FTD) had robbed me of my reasoning and made me act in a way that I was afraid of. I loathed myself in that moment. I was disgusted by actions.

As I continued to walk further into the dark snowy night, I heard a vehicle behind me, and someone was calling my name. It was a police canine van. Dawn had called the police and gave them my "Safely Home" number.

"Safely Home" is a nationwide program designed to help identify a person with dementia who is lost and assist in a safe return home. At all times I wear a bracelet with the inscription: "Mary Beth – Memory Loss – Call police."

It pulled up beside me and the officer tried to talk with me. I told him to leave me alone and I was fine. I continued to walk.

He persisted and I kept walking. Eventually he became sterner with me and I stopped. He asked me what was going on. In between my sobs, I told him I had FTD and I was only 46 years old. I told him that I had just yelled and screamed at my family. He brought it out of me that this is not who I was and that it was the disease.

After some talking, I eventually informed him that I would walk home. I did not want another cruiser to come and get me. I began trekking home following in my footsteps I had made only minutes before. I continued to cry. During all of this, my swallowing still bothered me. I kept spitting my saliva out of my mouth desperately trying to get rid of it. My house came into view.

Not only did I have the canine van following me, there was also a cruiser in my driveway. I continued to cry making my way into the open front door.

My family was there to greet me with open arms. I fell to my knees crying, saying, Dawn, It has started. The "it" I was referring to is this uncontrollable anger and being mean and hurtful to the people who I love the most. Brianna quickly put her arms around me, kept rubbing my back, and telling me how much she loved me. This went on for a bit. The police officer disappeared into the night.

My girls eventually got my coat and boots off and walked me to our bedroom. I crawled into bed.

During the entire time, my little girl, kept talking. It is not my fault; it is the disease. We don't quite know how to handle all of this, but we will get through it.

I do not know when Brianna grew up. At some time, my little girl became an adult. She laid beside me all the while soothing me with soft consoling words. My behaviour was embarrassing, and I kept telling her I was so sorry.

She then said it – *"MB – I love you unconditionally. You are the person who taught me what unconditional love is. Before you had entered my life, I had never even heard of the word."*

My eyes looked into her warm brown eyes. In a flash, I went back 10.5 years when I met Brianna. We had taken the basketball to a court and we were playing. My Brianna has grown up.

Unconditional love is extremely important to our family. When times have gotten tough, we remind each other, that we love them unconditionally. It is truly a love that has no bounds.

I am so proud of my girl. Parenting is a rewarding but can be difficult job. But I have taught something to Brianna that she now not only says but shows to me unconditional love.

Brianna has been thrust into a job role that she did not ask for. She has become my young care giver. There is not a job description to help guide her on what she should do in this position. She just does her best each day.

Since losing my license, Brianna has really stepped up and helps with the running of errands. She taxi's me to places I wish to visit. We have had a role reversal. I am now the one displaying the "terrible twos" and she is the one who is trying to manage my eradicate behaviour.

I am very scared about the pain and suffering I will bring to my family due to FTD. But I know in my heart, that my girls me love no matter what. No matter what this disease will bring, we will continue to love each other unconditionally.

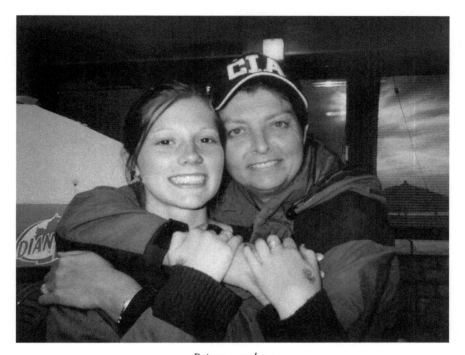

Brianna and me

Did I say how proud I am of my girl?

Gee Mom – I Don't Remember Either

Date: December 29th, 2012

Just recently I was introduced to an interesting terminology – sandwich generation. And no, it is not called that because I am part of a group who likes bologna sandwiches. Rather it defines those who are sandwiched between an ageing parent who needs help or care and their own ageing children. And for some condiments on this metaphorical sandwich, layer it with juggling jobs and family commitments. That's an awfully big sandwich!

This is a generation of caregivers, many of whom have elderly parents, aunts and uncles who have dementia. In fact, there are three million family caregivers in Canada.

My Mom is 83 years old and has Alzheimer's. My Dad is 86 years old and until four months ago, was her primary caregiver. Her care was greatly supplemented by my brothers and sister. At the end of August of this year, my parents moved from a beautiful apartment overlooking the St. Clair river to a Retirement Home. They love it.

I come from a large family. I have six brothers and one sister. I am the baby. Fortunately, for me, I was able to spend a great deal of time with my folks as my Dad had retired early and my Mom had stopped working. I developed a special bond with my Mom at a young age.

When it came time to truly address my Mom's memory loss, we called a family meeting. Therefore, it was of no surprise, that at this meeting I volunteered to discuss with Mom that she has dementia.

As I sat with my Mom holding her hand and looking into her blue grey eyes, I saw a lot of me. With tears in my eyes, Mom and I talked about her dementia. We held each other tightly without saying a word.

How strange it must have been for my brothers and sister to have to hold another family meeting, to determine how we were going to tell Mom and Dad about my dementia. It was decided that Debbie, Mark, and David would sit down with them and tell them the sad news. Dawn and I would visit them the next day after they had a chance to absorb the information.

I'm told that the conversation went as well as can be expected. What is most interesting is that my Mom asked some great questions: What does this mean for Mary Beth? And, will she move into the retirement home with her and Dad? She obviously understood.

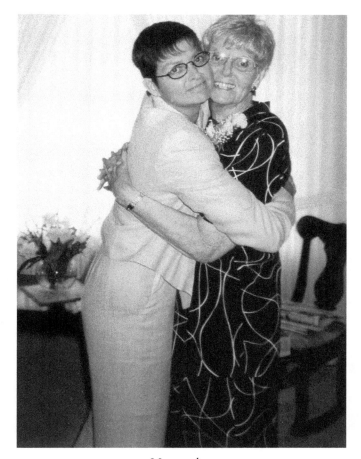

Mom and me

The next day, Dawn and I went to visit with Mom and Dad. My Mom kept hugging me and touching my face and smiling. It was a long time before she let me go. Mom's communication methods have changed since having Alzheimer's. She relies less on words and more on hugs. My family is enjoying those hugs very much.

Growing up, I used to get "Oh, you are just like Mom." We do have many of the same characteristics. Still, it seems a bit odd to be following my Mom's footsteps down into the world of dementia. Like Mom, I get up in the morning and eat a bowl of cereal or some porridge. And many times, I will go back to bed for a bit longer. I have developed quite a sweet tooth and my appetite, at times, does not seem to have much of a filter on it. Just like Mom. Now both Mom and I rely on my brother David to get us some wonderful Ravensburger puzzles. The number of pieces I can accomplish is a bit more than Mom. But not by much.

To bring us full circle, it's a funny thing to be part of the sandwich generation. Statistically, what are the odds of a living parent having dementia as well as a child?

What I don't know is the term for someone like Dawn. Only just turning 40, she is a caregiver for our daughter and me, her partner. And until recently, helped with my parents. Also, she has her own parents who are baby boomers and now into their 60's. Perhaps a definition is waiting to be labelled.

And yes, both Mom and I really do like bologna sandwiches!

YEAR TWO

Here we go Again

January 31st, 2013

Some days are easier than other days. Today, has not been easy. I had an appointment with my Geriatrician this morning. The last time I saw her was September 5th, 2012 when she diagnosed me with Frontotemporal Lobe dementia (FTD). I walked out of that appointment before it was finished. I did the same thing today.

When the appointment started, the Doctor told Dawn and I that we were there on the request of my family doctor. He was concerned about my aggressive behaviour.

About one week ago, we had a scary episode while in the car. While travelling in the evening back from Dawn's folks place, which is about an hour drive, something snapped inside me. There were four of us in the car – Dawn was driving, Brianna and her friend Shayla were in the back, and I was in the passenger seat. I knew something was going wrong and I told Dawn to get us home quickly.

No sooner had I said that, then the black cloud descended on me. I began to repeatedly hit with my closed fist the passenger window. This went on for a while. Dawn tried to talk me down, but I kept doing it. I than began to try and kick the front window. At some point, Dawn stopped the car and I was moved to the back seat with Brianna and Shayla took my seat. My eradicate behaviour continued and even escalated as I also started to yell obscenities out of the window.

I don't remember all of what happened but was told of my actions the next day. It lasted for about an hour. We were extremely lucky that

I did not cause a serious accident. Everyone was very shaken up by the incident. Bruising on my knuckles and hand had already begun.

I laid on the couch the entire next day. Not only was I feeling very tired, but also was extremely worried about the previous night. I had put my family in danger. This weighed heavily on me. I decided that I needed to find out if this was common for people diagnosed with FTD. I went up on a website forum I had recently discovered. This site is for people with FTD and their care givers. I began to search the entries to learn if others had experienced this before. Much to my relief and dismay, I found many entries about challenging behaviours of an FTD car passenger.

From what I could gather, a car ride can overstimulate someone with FTD. There were many suggestions by both parties on how to try and get around this stimulation. Some ideas were: move to the back seat; use ear plugs; don't have a radio on; put up a window shade; wear sun glasses; listen to Zen music, don't travel if tired, and take a mild sedative.

I shared this information with Dawn, and we strategized on how to help me be a safer passenger. We certainly were not the only ones to have this battle, as many experienced the same issue.

It was for this incident and some others, that I found myself sitting in front of the Geriatrician. She told us she was concerned about this behaviour. She also found it odd that I could share with her some of the strategies I found on the web. She thought that was unusual for someone with dementia.

I could feel the mood of the room change. She suggested to Dawn that if this happened again, that she should take me to the Emergency ward in the hospital to get evaluated by a psychiatrist. I could not believe she even said this out loud. Here we go again with the psychiatrists! I made a loud heavy sigh.

When we had started the meeting, she admitted that she did not know a lot about FTD as it is so rare. I piped up that it was found in 2% of all dementia. Since my diagnosis in Sept 2012, Dawn and I have learned a lot about this disease. I can tell you a great deal about its symptoms, the different variants, including diagnosing myself as bvFTD (Behavioural frontotemporal lobe dementia) based on my symptoms. This was not something that this doctor had done.

Dawn and I tried to tell the doctor that eradicate behaviour such as I had displayed, was common in bvFTD. The doctor kept with her suggestion to go see a psychiatrist if it should happen again. She also said that she would need help from other resources and mentioned Baycrest hospital in Toronto. Dawn replied that she had already contacted the hospital and our family doctor had been emailed the documentation necessary for the referral. We had done our homework.

Baycrest is the global leader in developing and providing innovations in aging and brain health. It has one of the few specialized programs, in the nation, to meet the individual needs of those with bvFTD. The program includes behaviour management techniques. Thankfully, Dawn has started the process to be referred to Baycrest.

Dawn and I have already been down the long and winding road of working with psychiatrists to help in healing me. We will not go back to that road as it is not the correct road. We will stay focused in moving towards the resources we believe can and will help us.

I realize today how incredibly important it is to not only be well-educated about FTD, but to also push back on individuals who we believe are not taking us on the right course of action. It is not that people are not trying to help, but rather that we do not agree with how they wish to help us. And that's O.K.

When putting together my team whose job it is to help me with my journey, I must have people onboard whose strategy I agree with. It is my right as a patient to decline treatment. If I am able, I will continue to look for the absolute best experts in their fields. It is critical for my team to have synergy and *listen* to me. After all, I am the patient.

A New Project

February 4th, 2013

Back in the day, I used to be a Sr. Business Analyst for a large well-known software company. This job afforded me wonderful opportunities of working with the very brightest and dedicated individuals across many global business units.

It seemed that my teams usually were given the most difficult projects with a higher percentage of possible failure rate. I was always amazed at how my team could take such a project and create and execute a solution. I felt fortunate to work with such intelligent, hard-working, and humble individuals. This team inspired me, and I earned something new every day.

Last week, I felt that excitement of starting a new project. Lisa, from MAREP, asked if I would be interested in being the editor for a yet to be defined or designed e-newsletter. It would follow along the same line, as the "By Us, For Us" MAREP booklets. The target audience will be people who have dementia and it will be created by the same. At this point, it is only an idea. Lisa needed someone to help drive the project. Yes, yes, yes! Sign me up.

After our meeting, I immediately jumped on the internet to see what was already out there. I fell into the trap of coming up with a solution, prior to understanding the requirements. I had to slow my jets down.

On the internet, I found an excellent document outlining the necessary steps titled, "How to Create an E-Newsletter: From Beginning to Send." I think this will help in providing the necessary framework to successfully accomplish the project.

To live well with dementia, it is important for me to seek out opportunities that will intellectually challenge me. I want to use my existing skills and even develop new ones. I believe this e-newsletter project will do just that.

If I had not partnered with MAREP, I believe that I would probably watch a fair bit of television today. Instead, I am looking forward to beginning the first steps of this exciting project. Not only will this help stimulate me, but it gives me a sense of accomplishment and contribution. It is that feeling that I look to embrace. I am off to live today as if it is my last. How exciting is that?!

You Can Have It – I Don't Need It Anymore

February 6th, 2013

Prior to the Anatomy Act of Ontario in 1843, there was not a legal process for the medical community to obtain corpses to be used for dissection or anatomy lectures in medical schools. Instructors had to rely on body-snatchers for cadavers. In the late 1870's, in Ontario, a cadaver could fetch $30 - $50. Thankfully, laws now regulate how a corpse can be obtained, and mirrors the need for necessary studies and research.

I have always been a firm believer in donating my organs and tissue upon my death. I have signed the back of my driver's license indicating this decision and have made my wishes known. Health Canada states one organ and tissue donor can save up to eight lives and help 75 more.

But I had never given it much thought about donating my brain. That was until I was diagnosed with Frontotemporal Lobe Dementia (FTD). Information that I read about this disease, indicates that at post-mortem the brain shows massive loss of nerve cells and considerable shrinkage. Scientists are working hard to understand this.

It is likely that there are several genetic changes that cause this disease. Research is concentrating on identifying changes on different genes on different chromosomes. For me, all this means is that there is no cure, but scientists are trying.

I asked myself, how can I help in obtaining a cure for this terrible disease? Upon research, I discovered a scientist who is a neuropathologist. She works at The Tanz Centre for Research in Neurodegenerative Diseases at the University of Toronto's Faculty of Medicine. She conducts autopsies and is a specialist in Alzheimer's. The Centre's website encourages people interested in participating in research on the causes of Frontotemporal dementia and other neurodegenerative diseases, to contact them. This includes brain donation.

So, I did just that. I contacted the Doctor. We had a brief conversation on the telephone. I told her I had FTD and would like to donate my brain. We will discuss "transportation" later. It was as simple as that.

Sometimes it is necessary and extremely important to discuss topics in which it makes people uneasy. I seem to have become more matter of fact about some of these topics. I have not been granted the luxury to decide on these things later. I must do it now – today. I do not know what tomorrow will bring. Neither do you – Reader. What are you waiting for?

If the donation of my brain helps just one person, then my gift to science has been well-worth it. I believe that my soul will leave my body upon my death and enter heaven. Therefore, I won't need my brain anymore. You can have it.

Your Loving Valentine

February 9th, 2013

St. Valentine's Day is one of my favorite holidays. I am not the roses and chocolate type of girl, but rather homemade cards, and a special dinner at home.

In our home, the feeling of love intensifies as February 14th draws near. Because of my fondness for traditions, I also have one for this marked day of love. Every year, I make my Valentine a homemade card professing my love. It is a tradition that My Girls have greatly enjoyed for the last 10 years.

My brother Mark has been making homemade Valentine cards for his Valentine, Mary Anne, for over 20 years. Mary Anne proudly displays these works of art, days before the big event. I'm always amazed at my brothers' talent, as every year he produces a new unique card. It is from him, that I have borrowed this idea.

Dawn keeps her Valentine Day cards, from me, in a special envelope. When you look at them, they reflect our 10-year relationship. Depending on the year, you may find a serious or funny card. Some of my cards are highly creative, whilst others not so much.

I have five days to create my card for this year. I have purchased some necessary art supplies. I have begun to think about possible ideas for this card. I believe this year, will be more of a serious one, once again professing my love and devotion. But we'll see how it all turns out on the Day.

I am incredibly happy to say that Brianna has now adopted this tradition of card making. Her young man of her choosing, is graced with a beautiful card made by her. I love it!

A few years ago, my Mom showed me a homemade card made by her Aunt Evelyne. It was to her and her younger brother Ron. It obviously meant a lot, as my Mom still has the card some 70 years later.

It is important to often express our love for each other. This does not mean if must be limited to our significant other. Since I have been diagnosed with Frontotemporal Lobe Dementia (FTD), I have told more people I love them then any time during my life. I don't want them to take it for granted.

Team Dementia – I love you. Happy Valentine's Day!

You CAN Teach an Old Dog New Tricks

Date: February 24th, 2013

The doorbell rang. I could see a tall figure holding a large box. My supplier was here. I opened the door and let him in. He had not been here for a delivery in a few weeks. We gave each other a warm hug and proceeded with pleasantries. I eyed the box and waited in anticipation for him to hand it to me. He slowly took off his boots. I continued to wait. We walked towards the kitchen where, finally, he gave me the box that held my supplies. I love that moment!

My supplier – is also known as my brother David. He is my puzzle supplier. If you like puzzles, then you can appreciate my anticipation. And if you don't, well, you are missing out!

David proceeded to tell me about the puzzles he had brought for me. He had a few of my favourite Ravensburger Puzzles. As the name suggests, this puzzle brand is made in Germany and shipped around the world. It is well-known for its high quality made from recycled board, they are strong, and the pieces properly fit together. This company has been in the puzzle business for over 100 years, so they know what they are doing. The pieces can range from just a few to 32,000 (the world's largest puzzle). That's a little too big for me. I keep to the range of about 60 – 180 pieces.

The second puzzle brand that David discussed with me is called Springbok. This company from the United Sates manufactures a line named "Puzzles to Remember" specifically for people with

Alzheimer's. The puzzle dimensions are the same as a 500 piece and contain adult themes. However, the pieces are much larger and range from 12 – 36. It too creates high-quality pieces allowing for easy interlocking. Although, it targets those with Alzheimer's, it is well-suited for someone like me who has dementia.

Growing up, my parents usually had a puzzle on the go. They enjoyed working together to complete it. Today, at the ages of 83 and 86, they still work together on puzzles and enjoy the satisfaction of finishing it. However, they stick to the Springbok Puzzles to Remember. Sometimes they receive help from my little nieces and nephews who also like a challenge.

This Christmas, my mother-in-law, Joyce, gave me a metallic 3D puzzle containing 36 pieces manufactured by Cheatwell. The extra challenge is not only is it 3D but that each piece is shaped in a square. How naive I was to think I could quickly finish this puzzle.

After opening the puzzle, I sat at the kitchen table with Nana, Dawn's grandmother and a.k.a. MB's puzzle companion. Nana and I have lots of chats about the latest puzzles we have been working on and periodically exchange them. We looked over this little tin box of 32 pieces. How hard could it be? Two hours later, we loudly told everyone just how hard it really was. People raised their eyebrows in disbelief.

During the 2 hours, Dylan, my young nephew of 10, causally picked up a few pieces of the puzzle, looked over the puzzle for a minute, then put them right into place. We couldn't believe it! Our eyes and brains obviously work very differently from this young whippersnapper.

In a day of technology, puzzles may seem a bit outdated to some people. Not to me. There are so many benefits of puzzles. They provide a great social setting for both the young and old, develop patience, focus and concentration. When you complete one, you have a wonderful feeling of success.

Oh yes, and of course they are fun.

For years, it was believed that our brain was "hard-wired" and our mental ability was fixed after childhood. But over recent decades, neuroscientists have discovered that brains are constantly changing. Growing new neurons and connections is a process called neuroplasticity. Change of the brain is associated with learning at the level of connections between neurons. New neurons can form, and existing synapses can change.

This is a hot topic in the world of research.

In layman terms, we must use it or lose it. For instance, did you use to know a foreign language? Haven't used it in a while? Now you can't remember it – because, you have not used it. Neuroplasticity suggests we have the ability to keep our brains sharp and capable of learning new skills well into our 90's. Like all organs, we must take good care of our brain and exercise it regularly by stimulation.

For those of us in Ontario, we are fortunate to have more than 500 neuroscientists in Ontario alone. Several important discoveries have positioned Canada as a global leader in the neuroscience market. Research groups are utilizing new technology and focus on top quality services. Baycrest Rotman Research Institute in Toronto is considered to have scientists that are probably the best in the world.

What does all this mean to me? I'm not a dog and I'm not old, but I can learn new tricks!

Sede Vacante

Date: February 28th, 2013

Today is a historical moment in the Catholic Church. Pope Benedict XVI prepares for his final day as the head of the Catholic Church. He has become the first Pope in 600 years to step down.

In his last speech to The General Audience of over 150,000 people, he stated, "...I have come to the certainty that my strengths, due to an advanced age, are no longer suited to an adequate exercise of the Petrine ministry." He will leave the Vatican for the last time and be brought to the papacy's summer retreat castle. The Swiss Guards who protect the pontiff, will march away and this will initiate the "sede vacante" - the empty seat of St. Peter.

Pope Benedict XVI's eight-year papacy will formally end.

My memory has drifted back to when I was a student in grade 4 at St. Benedict's school. My teacher, Sister Catherine, explained to my class the process of electing a new pope. She did an excellent job in communicating the significance of this holy and important event. Pope Paul VI had died in 1978. My grade four chums and I waited in anticipation for the new pope (John Paul I) to be announced.

In 1978, in Sarnia where I lived with my family, the Catholic Church for the most part followed closely to the rules and regulations involving altar boys. This was not the case for the church I attended – St. Benedict's. The parish priest, against custom, allowed girls to serve on the altar. I was fortunate to have the honour and the experience of being an altar girl.

It was a job which I took very seriously. I remember the feeling of being given my robe by Father Padelt. As I placed the long, white starched robe over my head, I felt like I was being transformed into someone else – someone much holier than myself. It was a blessing to be a part of the mass when the priest changed the bread and wine into the body and blood of Christ. I would carefully pour water over the priests' hands to ensure they were clean.

How different society is from my grade four days. I wonder how many people will even discuss today's historical event. Do Canadian's know that a potential replacement for the Pope is Canadian Cardinal Marc Ouellet of Quebec? If elected, he would be the first non-European pope.

I also wonder if Pope Benedict XVI is setting a new precedent. Individuals are living much longer than our forefathers. It is now normal to live into your 80's and even 90's. Will the new Pope live late into his life? At this age, will he be able to lead the Church? Or, will he too resign due to ill-health?

These are uncertain times. It will take a strong individual to take the helm of the Catholic Church and navigate it through these choppy waters. What words will people use to cross these waters? Are they words only meant for Catholics?

I believe that the "Golden Rule" does a wonderful job at conveying to all people the summation of Gods' entire way of life. The Golden Rule is: "In everything, therefore, treat people the same way you want them to treat you, for this is the Law and the Prophets." (Matthew 7:12). In 1993, 143 leaders from all the world's major faiths proclaimed the Golden Rule in the "Declaration Toward a Global Ethic" as the common principle amongst most religions.

Imagine if each person in the world adopted this as their personal motto. This one line can profoundly change the face of the world. These words can cross all cultures, political boundaries, ages, sexual orientation, religious affiliations, agnostic and atheists. Hmm... maybe a bit too John Lennonish?! *my fave*

My Dementia Team has people from a wide background and beliefs. At some later point in my life, I will be at the mercy of some of these individuals. I may look to them to help me get dressed, washed, and eat. They may have to help me in the basics of life. At that time, my voice may not be loud enough to be heard. I might not be able to vocalize my needs and desires. I truly hope that these members will have in their hearts The Golden Rule and act accordingly.

As Catholics look to the Vatican and wait for the words to announce a new pope: "Habemus Papam," I ask you to look into your own heart and ask yourself if you treat others as you would like to be treated. Only you know the truth. Only you and God.

My Unsung Hero

Date: March 3rd, 2013

It was all said by a box of Krispy Kreme donuts. Last night, Brianna (Bri) was at work at Walmart. She told Dawn that she was bringing home a surprise for me. Bri knows I like surprises. This morning when I went to make my coffee, I found my surprise on the counter. It was a box of Krispy Kreme donuts.

Of course, your first thought will be, "Isn't that thoughtful." For me, it is much more than that. That box of donuts represents Brianna's undying love for me. As I gave her a big hug and a kiss, my 18-year-old, transformed into a little girl of 7. She was that age when I met her for the first time. We were swimming at Laurel Creek park, and I would swim underwater towards her with my elbow above the water. I was pretending to be a shark. We laughed and I would do it again and again. Those were wonderful sun-filled days.

How quickly time has gone by. Brianna has grown up before my very eyes. We have gone through the trials and tribulations of growing from a young girl into a young adult. I still feel an immediate source of pride when I utter the words, "...my daughter."

Back in September of 2012, things immediately changed in our relationship. After the diagnosis of Frontotemporal Lobe Dementia (FTD), Brianna's responsibilities in the house changed. With my license being revoked, I look to Brianna to taxi me around to my appointments and pick up groceries. This is no easy task.

As my behaviour becomes more erratic, Brianna has learned to watch for warning signs. She now knows when I am becoming very tired to drive me home. Her learning has come at a high price for her.

Recently, we were out and about, and decided to go through a drive-through to get a hamburger. For some reason I become upset with Brianna and while in the drive-through told her to stop the car. I was getting out. Before Brianna had time to do anything, I opened the door of the car, and got out of the slowly moving vehicle. I stomped ahead and went into the building.

As I was placing the order for hamburgers, Dawn called me on my cell. I told her I was mad. Eventually, I came out with a bag of food and got into Brianna's car. We never said a word to each other. Later, I was told by Dawn how frightened Brianna was when I got out of the moving car. She did not see my go into the building and had no idea where I had gone. She called Dawn crying.

Last week, I heard an excellent analogy describing someone who has dementia. The analogy comes from Brydan (2005) who has had dementia for 10 years. She describes a beautiful swan gliding on the water while its legs are furiously paddling underneath. The beautiful swan above the water represents what most people see. It is those closest to me who can see me frantically paddling to stay afloat.

Brianna is sometimes "kicked" by my leg movements. She works extremely hard to support me in many ways. Sometimes, I notice these actions and tell her thank you, and other times, I do not.

Chris Wynn, whose Father had Alzheimer's disease produced a film titled: "Forget, Not Forgotten." This film shows the effects of the disease and the impact on caregivers. Chris is now working on another project which will focus on young people affected by the disease.

Later this month, Chris will be visiting our home to have an interview with Brianna. She will be one of the young caregivers featured in his new film. It should take about a year to make it. I wonder to myself if Chris is going to capture just the beautiful looking swan. Or, will there be clips of me paddling furiously while Brianna tries to support me.

I'm so proud of Brianna. Someday, when she reflects on these years, I hope she can remember how much I love her and appreciate her thoughtfulness.

The Red Cardinal

Date: March 11th, 2013

These last few days, I have had a touch of melancholy. I think its because of a combination of the long winter, the wet dreary days, and I've been fighting a cold. Some Canadians might also call this The Winter Blues.

As I was lying on the couch, debating whether to do research for my new MAREP project, I glanced out of the patio doors. It is a grey, rainy day. At the back of our large yard, something caught my eye near the bird feeder. A red cardinal flew to the feeder.

A smile crept onto my face. I thought about my brother Greg. He is brother number five in the lineup of eight children. That of course makes him my big brother. My big brothers have a great deal of responsibility: They need to keep their eye on me!

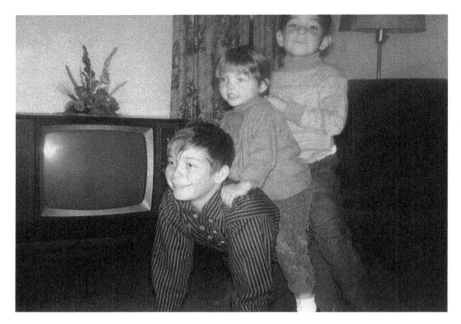

Greg, Me and David

My memories of Greg are all a caring, hardworking, loving man. One of my earliest memories of Greg is of him taking me skiing on a small hill with one skinny tree in the middle of it. Of course, the law of attraction had me ski right into the one tree! Greg came running down the hill to pick me up and wipe away my tears. That was it for skiing for me.

Greg always worked awfully hard to accomplish things. He encouraged me to do likewise. I could always count on him to give me some money for cleaning out his car. And there always seemed to be an apple pie from McDonalds for me to have when I was completed.

As we both grew older, he never stopped encouraging me to do my best at whatever I was doing. He helped me in making a big decision to go back to school to obtain a 3.5 years computer diploma. This shaped my life and led me to Toronto.

As I began to hit some of life's milestones, so did Greg. He met and married the love of his life, Margaret, and became a father to three children – Jason, Michael, and Kelley.

For years, I enjoyed being a big part of their weekends as Greg would have me come for a weekend visit. He showed me how to barbecue chicken, paint, garden and be a good example of a parent. He and Margaret shared with me the moment when I bought my first house. One that kept him busy helping to fix it up!

One month from today, Greg will have been gone for three years. After a brief and courageous battle with cancer, he died at the age of 54 years. I miss him.

About three years ago, just after Greg's passing, I began to have some bizarre experiences with a red cardinal in our back yard. For a good week, this black faced, red chested bird would land on the patio deck. It would hop along and would look directly at me. It was uncanny.

The red cardinal is a popular bird surrounded by superstition and considered to be a sign. The cardinals' red colour is symbolic of faith, so it can remind us to keep the faith when things look bleak. The cardinal call can cheer us up or cheer us on. It can be a symbolic sign of a deeply significant message for us.

Today, at my feeder, the little cardinals' red colour stood out against the backdrop of grey. For me, this beautiful bird represents Greg calling out to me. He's cheering me on, encouraging me to do my best. I hear you big brother. I am getting off the couch and I am off to seize the day for I can place no trust in tomorrow.

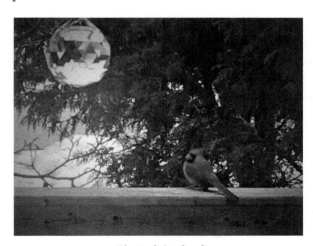

The Red Cardinal

Sugar Shack

Date: March 17, 2013

I'm a proud Canadian. Always have been. Always will be.

Rebecca is my new walking partner volunteer. The other day, we went for a walk on a country road across from our home. It was a beautiful day – sunny and the air was crisp. A perfect winter day.

As we hiked a long, I started to notice a familiar Canadian winter scene: maple trees with silver buckets hanging from silver spiels. My mouth immediately started to water. I could just imagine the yummy maple syrup being poured over a stack of steaming hot pancakes.

I am fortunate enough to live in a unique part of Ontario called Waterloo. It is the home to thousands of Mennonites of both the Old Order (horse and buggy) and the New Order. Maple Syrup season is a particularly active time for the Mennonites as they are busy collecting sap to make maple syrup. This in turn is sold from their country kitchen or the local market or to larger retailers.

One of the first times I went into a Mennonite kitchen was with Dawn and my Mom. We were there to pick out a bottle of maple syrup. There are different grades of syrup which the Mennonite woman educated us about. The lightest colored sap comes early in the season and is considered by many as the best. As daylight increases and temperatures warm, the concentration of sugars change. Syrup made from this sap takes on a darker colour. These are the light to amber classes. Finally, there is the dark class only to be sold for commercial use and it is considered less flavorful. In the grocery store, you usually only find the light-colored maple syrup. My favorite is the amber.

This means we usually make a trip to a local Mennonite farm to purchase a bottle. I always enjoy going to the farm and viewing and tasting the product of a lot of hard work.

This year, I think I would like to do something I haven't done in years. I would like to go to a Sugar Shack. A Sugar Shack is a small building where the sap collected from maple trees is boiled into maple syrup. On some farms, there are many activities for visitors to participate in such as a tour of the grounds, watching the process of boiling down the sap, and having a wonderful breakfast of pancakes and syrup.

A town near us, Elmira, hosts the world's largest one day maple syrup festival. It attracts nearly 70,000 people. For me, that is too many people as I would easily be overcome. We need to find a small venue.

A friend of Dawn's has a local farm and he taps his maple trees. He is positioned between a New Order Mennonite family on one side, and an Old Order Mennonite family on the other side. He works with these families to boil down the sap and make his maple syrup. Perhaps we could journey to there for an adventure.

I do not have a "bucket list" or a list of things I wish to accomplish before I die. However, since my diagnosis of Frontotemporal Lobe Dementia (FTD), I am more aware of things I would like to do. Visiting a Sugar Shack is one of them.

The time is ripe for the amber grade of maple syrup. My heart is filled with national and local community pride. The time is now to go off and enjoy the wonderful sights, sounds and tastes of a Sugar Shack. You know the old saying, "...live today as if it is your last, because you do not know what tomorrow will bring." Wish me well on my adventure.

We Do Not Have a Plan

Date: March 19, 2013

Last week, I received in the mail the requested pamphlets detailing Long-Term Care facilities found in the local region of Waterloo. I have been told by the medical experts that most likely I will eventually need to be placed in long-term care as it will be too difficult to take care of me.

I have Frontotemporal Lobe Dementia (FTD). I am 46 years old. Considering the mean of survival is eight years since diagnosis, I'm guessing a move is about four years away. But that's all it is – a guess.

I have asked my Case Manager to sit down with Dawn and I and work with us in developing a plan designed to keep me at home if possible and out of an institution. In my naivety, I did not realize what a difficult request I have made.

At the same time of my inquiry for a plan of my own, I have begun to do some research on Canada's National Dementia plan. Some of you may be puzzled by this. That's because you know that Canada does not have a national plan for dementia. Let me say that again more slowly –

*Canada **DOES NOT** have a national plan for dementia.*

The Alzheimer Society of Canada and its provincial chapters have done a good job at informing Canadians the statistics surrounding the "dementia tsunami." I know that in 2011, a new case was diagnosed every 5 minutes. I have read the recent report commissioned by the Alzheimer Society titled: "Rising Tide: The Impact of Dementia on Canadian Society."

If you have not read it, you should. It will scare you. The up-to-date statistics and costs associated to dementia is simply staggering. As of 2011, the following countries have established national dementia plans: Australia, England, France, Republic of South Korea, Netherlands, Norway, Scotland, and Wales. Canada has yet to do so or make dementia a national priority.

In my quest for knowledge, I turned to a web site called: Dementia Support Networks. A Meeting of the Minds. On it is the topic of a National Dementia strategy for Canada. This is an interesting and informative presentation. With that said, I am very much concerned about the basis of what the national plan will be made on.

Here it is:

• Improving skills and training of health-care workers and family doctors who are pivotal in the early diagnosis and provision of care throughout the disease.
• Bringing research funding in line with cancer and other chronic conditions to find ways to prevent dementia and find a cure.
• Supporting family caregivers.

- Increasing awareness of the importance of prevention and early intervention.
- Building an integrated system of care.

Do you see anything missing? If not, read the five bullets again. Or better yet, read it from my perspective – someone who has dementia.

It does not say anything about a person with dementia! It talks around it but not to it. I'm still here. I just happen to have dementia. I can still understand and want to be involved in my own plan of care. I cannot take things for granted and assume the basis of this plan will take care of me.

Canada needs a national dementia plan – now. The provinces need a dementia plan – now. Thank you to all who are working hard to help drive towards a plan. I honestly believe in the power of the people. Readers, it is the time to push our policy makers. Do not sit back and assume someone else will do the work. We need you.

Who will Carry the Baton?

Date: March 24th, 2013

I love history. I gravitate towards individuals who were/are instrumental in fighting for a just cause. Names like Rosa Parks, Terry Fox, Martin Luther King, Gandhi, Eleanor Roosevelt, Mother Theresa, Nelson Mandela, and Michael J. Fox are a few examples of beacons of strength and represent change.

It is exceedingly difficult to change status quo. The names previously mentioned did not invest one day of their life to reform. Rather, they embraced change at any given moment.

This week, I have been searching for advocates who have dementia. I wish to reach out to them, listen to their words of wisdom and be inspired by them. Unfortunately, they are few and far between.

By the very nature of dementia, it is that much more difficult to speak, remember, and write. Years of prejudice, stigma and lack of education are huge barriers to altering our current state of affairs. I visualize a mountain with a line of advocates, with dementia, nearing the peak. And when the leader reaches the peak, she raises her hands in triumph. But then, she looks out and discovers this is only one mountain in a huge range. My advocate turns to the line following her, and she cheers them on and congratulates them for reaching the top. Without skipping a beat, she says... only a few more mountains to climb.

Since my diagnosis of Frontotemporal Lobe Dementia (FTD), I have added names to my list of people I admire, for their efforts to initiate change in the world of dementia. Individuals such as Brenda Hounam, Carl Wilson, Kate Swaffer and Jim Mann are amongst them. With the assistance of others, they have forced change for those with dementia to live well.

I worry about what will happen to this movement when the leaders are no longer able to do so. Who will pick up the baton and run with it? We need to be less of a single line and more shoulder to shoulder in our numbers and formation. This is by no means an easy task.

I have been struggling this week with my memory. My daily games of Mah-jong have been more difficult. I have not been finishing my brain exercises at Luminosity as they have been too challenging. For a split minute, I had forgotten how to make hamburgers and defrost meat. I am frustrated.

When these things happen, I wonder how much longer it will be until I can't remember it at all.

I sometimes feel the pressure of urgency. I know I am capable to help in education, to fight against stigmas and to push for government policy changes. The limelight does not scare me because I believe I understand what needs to be done. It needs to be done - now – while I still remember and can speak and write.

My niece, Jennifer, did something significant for me this week. She sent an email to a government Minister pleading for funding to be allocated in the 2013 budget and for the creation of a national dementia plan. Further to that, she emailed TVO's Producer of The Agenda. Her email said: "I wonder if your show might be interested in Canada's lack of a dementia plan as a potential topic. I'm sure my aunt would be honoured to be in touch with you. She is an extremely bright woman and engaging speaker."

A short few hours later the Producer of The Agenda, responded to Jen's email. She thanked Jen for her suggestion and asked how to get in contact with her or I. I do not know what, if anything, will happen with TVO. But it is the provision of an opportunity to fight for a national dementia plan that is to be recognized.

My other niece, Heather, also provided an opportunity for me to be heard. Heather twitted a link to my speech on Living Well with Dementia on You Tube. The great thing is Heather has 504 people following her. That is a wide audience! I can only hope that at least a few people are curious enough to click on the web-link and watch my speech.

It is important for people with dementia to do the best they can every day. Likewise, it is also important for others to help support us in our fight. I cannot let the baton drop. We still have many mountains to climb before the land of milk and honey is to be reached.

I searched the internet for some inspiring words to close out my journal. Interestingly, they are about Rosa Parks, who had dementia but was known for her civil rights activism. Mia Bay, Professor of History and Director of the Center for Race and Ethnicity, Rutgers University, provides words to live by: "Rosa Parks' story tells us you don't have to always have been a leader to do something important and to make an impact, and you don't have to be a big personality or a loud person to take a stand. You can be a quiet person of principles, and these quiet people who work behind the scenes are important to social change."

I Have a Worm in my Ear?

Date: March 26th, 2013

Do you ever get that song stuck in your head that just keeps playing over and over? I do. It happens to me a lot.

Yesterday, while watching CBC news, there was a segment on this phenomenon. These mental tunes are nicknamed "earworms." You learn something new every day!

For about the last year, I have started to sing to myself – or to my dog, Shiloh. I can assure you; I was never much of a singer. But things have changed. I often catch myself doing this and sometimes I even add in a few dance steps to accompany the music.

My repertoire ranges the gamete. Right now, some of my favorite tunes are:

♫ Tweet tweet, twiddle twiddle, there's only one candy with the hole in the middle (Life Saver
commercial)
♫ Lord of the Dance – Church song written by Sydney Carter
♫ I'm Gonna Be (500 Miles) – The Proclaimers
♫ Sugar, Sugar – The Archies, and
♫ Oompa Loompa by Willie Wonka.

I'm told that I even sing in my sleep! Dawn has said that I can break out in a resounding rendition of "Row row row your boat."

I must confess that my very favorite song to sing comes from Mary Poppins: supercalifragilisticexpialidocious! I have long lost count of how many times I have watched a video singing along with Mary Poppins.

My audience of one, Shiloh, never seems to tire of me singing and clapping to a song.

What is interesting is that my Mom, who has Alzheimer's, also loves to watch the same music video over and over. On any given day, she can watch The Celtic Thunder for hours, never seeming to tire of it. I'm not sure my Dad feels the same way.

Some of the ritualistic behaviours of Frontotemporal Lobe Dementia (FTD), includes clapping and singing. I think it is obvious I am now displaying these behaviours. Of all the different kinds of behavioural changes I might show; I figure this one isn't too bad.

The human body is susceptible to many types of worms – pinworms, roundworms, hookworms and tapeworms. Although, we generally don't associate these parasites with humans currently. I just must face the facts that I now have an earworm.

If you catch me singing, please feel free to join in. And don't worry, you don't have to be in key, because I'm certainly not!

Self-portrait

Date: April 2nd, 2013

Several years ago, I was fortunate enough to visit the van Gogh museum in Amsterdam, The Netherlands. I have always been a fan of Vincent van Gogh's paintings. They seem to be able to draw out a strong emotional response. At the top of my favorites list includes "Joseph Roulin" (The Postman), "The Potato Eaters", and "Self-portrait", 1889.

van Gogh painted many self-portraits. In fact, between the years 1886 and 1889, he painted himself 37 times. I wonder why he did that. He battled frequent bouts of mental illness. Perhaps as he went through these bouts, he saw a different man in the mirror each time. Thus, the need to paint himself again and again.

My last few days, I seem to be struggling with remembering things that just happened a few hours before. For instance, I thought today I had a nap for one hour. Dawn told me it was three hours and not one. How can I not know that? Yesterday, I sent a detailed email to someone. Today, I kept rereading the email as I was surprised at how articulate it was.

There is a great deal of discussion and research on people, who have dementia, who develop extraordinary new artistic abilities. Individuals who never even had an interest in art, find the urge to paint. As language abilities erode, the visual sense becomes more precise. Incredible paintings done by people having dementia can be found on the internet, ready for sale.

I have yet to pick up a paint brush. My current new talent is writing. I never did it before and now look at me! I have tapped into some part of my brain that has been rarely used and is not damaged. At some point, I hope I do start to paint. There are all kinds of wonderful side effects.

I like the idea of creating a piece of art to be hung on a wall with pride. If I do begin to paint, I wonder if I will create a self-portrait. Or perhaps, like van Gogh, I will create many self-portraits.

If I painted 37 pictures in three years like he did, how will they change? I almost want to create one, now. I would use this picture as the base of comparison. As my frontotemporal lobe dementia (FTD) worsens, I will continue to paint self-portraits. What will my last portrait look like in comparison to my first portrait? Will I recognize the woman in the self-portrait?

I wonder.

What Do You Do?

Date: June 5th, 2013

In a conversation with a person you have just met, it is common to ask the individual what she does for a living. I find this question to be awkward. What should I say? I am sick – I don't work? I have dementia. I am disabled. None of your business?

I'm sure you can see my dilemma. I ask myself, *why* do I find the question awkward? The reason is because I have been raised with the Protestant Work ethic. From a young age, I was taught that it was important to work, and it gave me a sense of pride. Today, because I have Frontotemporal Lobe Dementia (FTD) I do not work and therefore, the feeling of pride has left me.

My first job was that of a T.V. Guide delivery girl. I was probably about 9 years old. I had a little white shoulder bag with the books in it. I would hike up and down our street and give people their guides. This job has obviously gone the way of the dinosaur! But I'll always remember the source of pride it gave me and the feeling of the jingling coins in my pocket.

It seems that I always had a job. One time, while I was playing basketball in my driveway, a real estate agent approached me asking if there where any boys in the neighbourhood. He explained he was looking to hire someone to cut the grass of a house that was for sale. Being confident in myself, I asked him why does it need to be a boy? I could cut the grass – no problem! He chuckled, and said I was hired. I'm thinking I was about grade six when this happened. Once again, I was looking for the jingling coins in my pocket.

As I grew older, life would eventually lead me to Toronto for my new job in computers. In 1994, the world of internet had yet to be taken mainstream. Those were the days of faxing. I was hired to be technical support for a new Canadian product called WinFax. I was one of five girls on the floor of about 80 technicians. I experienced prejudice as people wanted to speak to a "real" technician – not a woman. At the time, this company was the leader in its field of technology. It was an exciting company to work for. As I moved up the ladder, the expectation for me to travel increased. It was common to receive a telephone call and be asked to be in California for the next day. For about two years, I commuted back and forth from Toronto to California. I was asked to relocate to the States, to live in Oregon or California. I declined because of my national Canadian pride.

Before leaving the company after 10 years, I had the great fortune of travelling, for work, to the following countries:

- ✈ Argentina
- ✈ Brazil
- ✈ Mexico
- ✈ France
- ✈ Germany
- ✈ Ireland
- ✈ The Netherlands
- ✈ Italy
- ✈ Switzerland
- ✈ United States
- ✈ United Kingdom
- ✈ South Africa
- ✈ Republic of Singapore
- ✈ Australia

My next position was that of us being co-owners in an engineering recruiting company. It is a story of disappointment and failure. Nothing I am proud of. That's the way life sometimes goes. It is here when I started to display signs of FTD and, ultimately, I was put on a leave of work from my doctor. Thus, the beginning of the question: What do you do for a living?

It has taken me four years to get here, but I now know what to say: "I'm retired." To me, the definition of retirement includes working for most of your life and then stopping usually at an older age. I meet one of the two criteria. The fact of it is, I will not live to an older age, so that criterion does not apply to me.

It's interesting the games our mind can play on us. Simply by thinking and stating "I'm retired" I have a new sense of ease about me. I do not fill guilty anymore for not being part of the 9-5 crew. I eat two bowls of ice-cream instead of one. I do not let the clock dictate my day.

Ultimately, this means I do not have to state the dreaded word "disabled."

I really have worked for most of my life. I have wonderful and great accomplishments to be proud of. The world-wide experiences have been most gratifying and educational. But the fact is the fact. It feels GREAT to be retired! Oh, and one more thing to add, although I'm only 46 years old, I'm starting to get grey hair. I fit in with the retirees, simply fine.

The Raising of the Barn

Date: April 17th, 2013

Yesterday, was an exciting day here at our home. Just after 9:00 am, the doorbell rang, and in came some of my family members. Kisses and hugs were given to Jan (sister-in-law), Joe (brother-in-law), Mark (brother) and David (brother). They came with boxes filled with paint cans, brushes, and an assortment of other tools.

It all started a few weeks ago, when I asked David for assistance in painting our family room. It is something in which he excels in. He responded by saying that there were a group of them coming to lend a hand. And yesterday was when it all happened.

The group quickly organized themselves and planned the strategy on how to tackle the objective. Before I knew it, the paintbrushes were quickly changing the wall colour. Each person has their own individuals' strengths which was capitalized on by the group. Together, it was a well-oiled painting machine!

Conversation was free and some gentle bantering was done. This in combination with some food and drink made for a wonderful, productive day. At 3:00, good-byes were said, and the group piled into the car and headed off to their individual homes. Mission accomplished.

When I reflect on the day, I realize we had partaken in a modern-day version of "barn raising." For you younger folks, a barn raising describes a collective action of a community, in which a barn for one of the members is built or rebuilt collectively by members of the community. Barn raising addressed the need by enlisting members of the community, unpaid, to assist in the building of their neighbours' barns. Because each member was entitled to recruit others for help, the favour would eventually return to each participant.

I must say, the pioneers really had a good thing going with barn-raising. There are so many benefits generated by yesterdays events. For us, we felt a sense of accomplishment of painting a room of professional quality, all within a few short hours. We learned from each other, tricks of the trade. It was fun! It strengthened our personal bonds. And, we know we are there for each other, if another "barn" needs to be raised.

Being the youngest of a family of 8 children, has its benefits. Many a time, I have been introduced as "this is my baby sister." This still happens! Since being diagnosed with Frontotemporal Lobe Dementia (FTD), I have reached out to my family for support.

As unique as they are as individuals, so too is the way each family member contributes to my wellbeing. On any given day, along with thoughts and prayers, I may receive emails, cards, telephone calls, presents, visits and videos. All of which raises my spirit and which I deeply appreciate.

An old friend, of whom I lost contact with, reached out to me after hearing I was sick. She commented to me "I was quite pleased to learn when reading the various journals that you seem to have remained close to your brothers and sister. So many families that I know are not so lucky." It made me think. I AM lucky. In a day and age of technology, long-distance and crazy schedules, barn-raising has gone by the wayside. How unfortunate. It takes time, effort, and desire to build and maintain our family relationships.

As I forge ahead on my journey of dementia, I will continue to rely on my family members to give me strength in their own individual ways. The next time a barn needs to be raised, I will bring my tools of expertise, and help in contributing to my family's collective goal. How fortunate I am to be a Wighton.

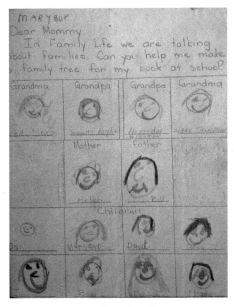

Wighton family

Earth Day

Date: April 21, 2013

Every so often, an event comes along forcing me to stop concentrating on myself and look at things from a global perspective. Today is one of those events.

The sound of birds chirping woke me up today. Much better than an alarm clock! I have taken my coffee to the family room where I can watch the hungry finches eating their Niger seed breakfast. The sun is just starting to make its appearance. It is going to be a glorious Earth Day 2013. Earth Day is an annual day on which events are held worldwide to demonstrate support for environmental protection. It is celebrated in more than 192 countries every year. This is truly a spectacular event created by the power of the people. A grass-roots effort, this Day was created by concerned individuals who fought for wider recognition and organization. Well done!

Living in Kitchener, Ontario, I wish to toot my own horn. Millions of people around the world practice source separation using the "Blue Box". Kitchener has the honourable distinction of launching the first ever Blue Box program on September 17th, 1981. Today, more than 650,000 tonnes of secondary resource materials are diverted by Ontario households through the blue box program. And as they say, the rest is history.

Having been diagnosed with Frontotemporal Lobe Dementia (FTD), I tend to look at things in a boundary of time. I know I will not live into my 80's. It is that much more important to seize the day and place no trust in tomorrow.

Today, I intend on picking up garbage along the roadside on Kraft Drive. This beautiful country road is where I walk. Unfortunately, it has some garbage beside it, probably due to the wind blowing out garbage from blue boxes. This small act will combine with millions of others small acts, and ultimately produce a strong effort in reducing waste in the world.

It is extremely important we act as mentors to our children. This can also be known as "putting your money where your mouth is." I must lead by example to reduce, reuse, and recycle.

Off I go to seize the beautiful, sunny filled day. I hope you join me.

A Love Story

Date: April 30th, 2013

Throughout history, love has found its way to certain couples, for which they have become famous. Some of my favourite lovers include: John Lennon and Yoko Ono, Cleopatra and Mark Anthony, King Edward VIII and Wallis Simpson, Grace Kelly and Prince Rainier III, and Queen Victoria and Prince Albert.

To my list, I'd like to add one more couple, who are not known world-wide, but certainly are in my books: Helen and Bill Wighton. Now you can argue that I'm prejudicial, and I suppose there is some truth in that. However, when you look at this relationship, it possesses all the characteristics of the other larger-than-life couples.

But, before I get into that, let me first introduce you to Helen and Bill – my Mom and Dad. It was June 24th, 1950 in Sarnia Ontario. After two years of courtship, Helen Moran and William Wighton exchanged vows of love and commitment through thick and thin. And so, began the love story of over 63 years of marriage for this dashing young couple.

Dad was already working at Imperial Oil and Mom was a legal secretary. Before they knew it, Mom was pregnant with their first child, Dan. Soon, the young family would move into a new home on Superior Street. As the couple continued to have more children, Dad continued to add additions to the house. In 1966, the couple rounded out their family with me. In total there were eight children: Dan, Jim, Bob, Debbie, Greg, Mark, David, and me.

I can't imagine how difficult it must have been to keep a healthy, loving relationship in such a busy home. Although, I always saw the signs of it. Dad is quite the dancer. On numerous occasions he would sweep Mom from her kitchen chair and whirl her about. It brought them back to the days of dancing to Tommy Dorsey and Glen Miller at Kenwick-on-the-Lake. This is where they first met.

Life for the Wighton's has had its high's and lows, like most marriages. The backbone of the marriage is their deep faith, coupled with mutual respect and unconditional love.

Today, marks one of the last chapters in their lives. Mom's health has been declining. She will move to a long-term care facility without Dad. Within the month, he will move into the same facility but in the retirement section. They will no longer share a bedroom as they have for the last 63 years. With the love of his life on his mind, Dad had to make an incredibly hard and unselfish decision. Mom will get the best care possible regardless of his own potential loneliness.

Since being diagnosed with Frontotemporal Lobe Dementia (FTD), I have seen my own relationship with my love, Dawn, go through many acts of unselfishness.

I am extremely fortunate and blessed to have this special couple as my parents. It has provided me with a wonderful example to which I can base my own relationship.

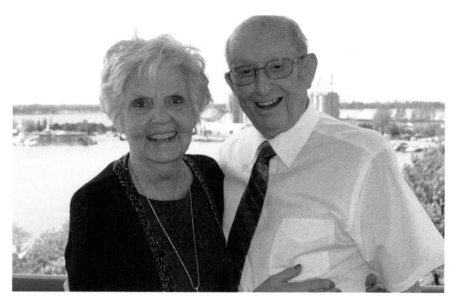

Helen and Bill Wighton

In a few hours, Mom will be in her new home. In Dad's mind, he probably will be thinking the famous Winnie-the-Pooh quote: "If you live to be a hundred, I want to live to be a hundred minus one day, so I never have to live without you." Just like he has done all their marriage, I have an inkling Dad will bring her flowers. Because that's what the great lovers do.

Names Will Never Hurt Me?

Date: May 6th, 2013

The longer I am sick with Frontotemporal Lobe Dementia (FTD), the more times I encounter stigma and prejudice. It has made me take a step back and review my own actions and possible prejudices. I realize that for as long as the world has been alive, so has stigma. I wonder why. What makes us intolerant to others who are different from ourselves?

At a young age, I was taught the childhood phrase: "Sticks and stones will break my bones, but names will never hurt me." It seems that humankind has not yet advanced past name calling. The rhyme was to be used while I was under attack by someone who was saying mean things to me. The problem was the names still hurt – even when I was putting on a brave face.

This past week, I experienced a frontal attack of hurtful comments. On a website, who's audience is those with FTD and carers, a post was made by a carer. This person and her children have been living for 17 years with her husband who has FTD. She described her journey with her husband and that they will be relieved when he dies. When he dies, no one will miss him. One of the children said, "Dad has lived past his expiration date."

I do not know what it is like to live with someone who has FTD. I just know what it is like to live with FTD. I have not walked in the shoes of that family – only my own. I cannot imagine the pain they have experienced of losing their loved one. I just know the pain I experience feeling me slip away from my own family. I can't imagine how scared they must be – I just know how scared I sometime am.

We choose hurtful words in response to our pain, anger, grief, and sorrow. When doing this, the pain just continues to intensify as more people are hurt.

When I said out-loud, "...lived passed his expiration date" I realized how the phrase "sticks and stones will break my bones, but names will never hurt me" is untrue. Names do hurt me. The word "expiration" is used in connection with milk, meat, or other preserves. It is not a word to be associated with the death of a human.

Dawn and I talked about this incident and we both vocalized our bruised feelings. Dawn responded to this post. Her words were in defence of me and others with FTD who cannot vocalize for themselves. Unfortunately, this led to others also using similar hurtful words to describe their relationship with someone with FTD. This battle will not be won by anyone.

I do not understand why we choose to hurt each other. What I do know is kind words are like a salve to me. They help in soothing my aching heart. Kind words are inexpensive and easy to distribute. What better medication is there?

Wheels

Date: May 9th, 2013

I started driving when I was 17 years old. I loved it. It gave me such freedom and made things much easier driving to and from work. Much better than my bicycle.

While I was travelling for work, I usually stayed for at least one week and so I would rent a car. It allowed me to come and go as I wished. I also took advantage of seeing the sites in my free time. In some countries, driving was a little more challenging. In Australia and Ireland, you must drive on the "wrong side" of the road. In Costa Rica, I had to drive a 4-wheel drive as the rain forest roads were very rough.

One of the most unnerving roads I drove on, was in Ireland along the Cliffs of Moher. As I drove white knuckling the stick-shift on the "wrong side" of the road, I was distracted by the cliffs that rose some 700 feet above the ocean. My passengers kept encouraging me to go faster than 3rd gear, but I was reluctant. Nature has a great way to keep the speed limit down for those speed demons.

Closer to home, I was the dedicated driver for the family. It was a responsibility which I enjoyed. But it was two years ago, when I started to experience some challenges navigating through the city that I live in. I got lost in our subdivision and found it hard to remember how to get to some places. As I drove, road signs would come at me and I didn't always know which way to turn. It was unnerving.

Although I knew something was cognitively wrong, I didn't want to tell anyone for fear of what may happen. That fear was realized when I was told that I had Frontotemporal Lobe Dementia (FTD). The second point the doctor stated was that I couldn't drive anymore - effective immediately. Sometimes, I play that moment in my mind in slow motion. At that time, it was just as devastating news as the disease. It felt like someone punched me extremely hard in my stomach. In a flash, I saw my independence leave me. I was angry and disbelieving. I was told that although I do not get lost as easily as someone with Alzheimer's, my ability to make sound judgement and process different stimuli was compromised.

I have always been an independent person. I'd rather not ask for help if I can avoid it. Without a license, I am now forced to ask for help. Taking a city bus could prove too challenging and possibly overwhelming. I'm at the mercy of others. This is not something I like. Thankfully, my family and friends taxing me around does not seem to be too much of a burden.

Yesterday, was the first real day since my diagnosis, that I was very bothered about not having a license. I wanted to drive to different stores and browse. I didn't want someone to hold my hand and cart me around. I felt like a child. I was angry.

What is important to know is that I believe the doctor made the correct decision. If I'm an unsafe driver than I should not be allowed to drive. Period.

My 86-year-old Dad has written the mandatory driving test for people over 80. He passed it and was pleased as it affords him continued independence. I must admit I was a bit jealous. I too wanted that independence. Once that feeling passed, I am now happy for my Dad.

As the tsunami wave of those with dementia approaches, so too will thousands of individuals experience my pain of having their license revoked. It is said the number of drivers with dementia in Ontario will more than double from about 45,000 today to nearly 100,000 in 2028.

Our population continues to age. Ontario's transportation ministry is busy discussing possible changes targeting this ageing group. Possible on-road testing; graduated licensing and de graduated licenses are all possible. It is a contentious issue.

My hope is that while the transportation ministry is busy planning for this wave, so too are families. Challenging discussions will have to had with loved ones. It is difficult to ask someone to give up their independence.

Wheels. How I miss them.

Camping

Date: May 23rd, 2013

Camping has been part of my life beginning at a young age. My folks used to pack us kids up and head down river to some campgrounds. We had a small trailer with the basics and tents for the older kids. It felt like we were in a different world. I loved the freedom, campfires, and fishing.

My older siblings tell great tales of homemade trailers, wheels flying off, leaky tents, and Mom praying in the front car seat that we will all be O.K. It doesn't matter how many times I hear the same stories; they still make me laugh as I imagine the chaotic scenes.

My own family has also enjoyed camping – although we prefer to purchase our trailers rather than build one. I remember the first time it rained while we were in our new trailer. I felt like a queen as I looked out the window at the poor campers in rain-soaked tents. I hugely appreciated the warm and cozy environment. I have many wonderful memories.

Last week, we parked our trailer for the season up near Southampton. It is on a beautiful mature campsite in a lovely campground. As enjoyable as it was, it was a bit strange for us. This was the first time we were doing it without Brianna. She now has responsibilities at work and needs to be there. She will come up to visit for a few days when she is able.

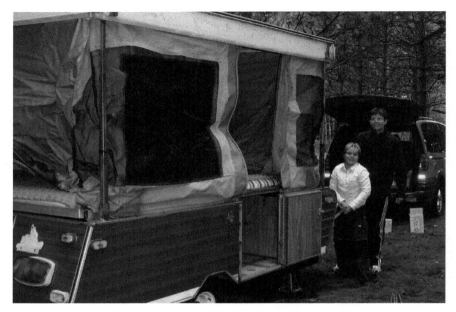

Brianna and me – "The little trailer that could"

Life is a constant change. Although camping is in my blood, it has changed with who, when, where and how long I have camped. This is just one more change.

As I walked my dog, Shiloh, on one of the trails, I reflected on how lucky I was. The birds were chirping, the sun was warming me, and I felt at peace with the world. Dawn and I were embracing life and the adventures that come with it. Just because I have dementia, does not mean I don't want to get out of the house and live. I do! Sure, maybe we need to adjust a few things, but that's O.K. This is about living life with dignity and carpe diem (that old Latin saying about living life to its fullest and place no trust in tomorrow).

As we worked on making our trailer ready and homey for the season, we watched a pair of robins create a bird's nest. They were busy just like us. Both birds were whizzing back and forth with twigs in their mouths. We all eyed each other completing our work. It was truly something to watch.

There is much to be said about being outdoors and having dementia. There is evidence of the benefits of green exercise (physical activity out in nature) and dementia. There is an interesting company in the U.K.

whose focus is connecting people with dementia to nature and a sense of adventure. Some of their holidays include sailing and canal boat holidays.

What a wonderful method to help in making memories for both the person with dementia and carer. We will be spending a great amount of time at our trailer. We are making a concerted effort to go out and live and be game for adventures. I'm excited for this. I may not remember everything, but it won't stop me. Besides, we can always take pictures!

Silver & Gold

Date: May 28th, 2013

I am emerging from a weeklong "FTD funk." This is what I have termed as a Frontotemporal Lobe Dementia (FTD) induced mental fog. Symptoms of this disease such as lack of motivation, apathy, irritability, forgetfulness, poor decision making and difficulty in word finding descended upon me and warped my clear thinking – just like fog.

While in this fog, I realized what was happening. It is hard to describe it to someone who has not experienced it. I reached out to a new friend who has dementia. In my email, I described to her my frustration with this fog. It was interesting, because just by writing to her, I felt a bit better. Her response with words of wisdom and an offer to be a sounding board helped in clearing my head.

This once again has reminded me of the importance of friends – young or elderly, new, or old. When I was first diagnosed, my sister told me how I would meet new people who would help me in my journey. The wisdom of my older sister has proven true.

I am reminded of a childhood song: "Make new friends but keep the old, one is silver, the other is gold." I remember asking my Mom what this ditty meant. She described it something like this: it is saying that new friends are valuable, like silver and old friends are a great treasure, like gold. Don't lose your old friends to new ones.

In the last four months, two old friends wished to reconnect with me. Remarkably, they both googled my name on the internet and discovered I have a terminal illness. They reached out to me to tell me of their support for me. One even confessed to me that my Mom made the best butter tarts she has tasted. That's a true friend!

I am truly fortunate to be blessed with the friends I have. I have enjoyed deep and meaningful relationships where I do not wear a heavy coat of armour. My relationships are respectful, comforting, and supportive. Over the years, I have developed numerous friendships. Many of these relationships have fallen by the wayside. However, I have wonderful memories of those times. They have impacted me and have contributed to shaping who I am.

As you might imagine, FTD can be hard on my relationships. It is widely known that due to its symptoms some friends may disappear. Because of that, I find it extremely important to educate people about the disease and my state of well-being. I hope that it will help ease friend's potential discomfort when speaking with me.

For some special friends, FTD is instrumental in developing yet another level of degree of friendship. Today, I will be attending a funeral. It is for a good friend of my in-laws who died in a motorcycle accident. This shocking death once again served as reminder of living for the day. He will not have said his goodbyes and ensured all were well with his friendships. He will not have had the opportunity to ensure things were in good order.

I do have the opportunity. It is something which is especially important to me. My dear old friends – I love you.

My new friends – love you, too. And to both, thank you for taking this journey with me. You are a good friend.

The Long Hallway

Date: May 31st, 2013

The smell of urine has not left me.

Yesterday, Dawn decided for us to visit a long-term care facility. At 2:00 p.m. we arrived at a nice-looking building. I sat on an outside bench trying to absorb what we were about to do. We were here to have a tour looking to access if this could be a suitable place for me to one day live at.

It started last week, when my case worker from CCAC gave me the necessary paperwork to fill out for submitting my preferences for long-term care. Having Frontotemporal Lobe Dementia (FTD), I will eventually require a great deal of care. It is our hope that I will always remain in our home. We will hire necessary workers to assist Dawn. Our home will be modified to accommodate my changing needs: bathroom renovations, wheelchair ramp, stair lift, etc.

However, it is also important for us to have a "plan b." If I do require more care than is manageable at home, I must have my ducks-in-a-row. This means, having my name on a waiting list for up to three long-term care facilities. The search has begun.

Yesterday, marked the first visit of a potential home. From the exterior, the building seemed quite nice. Lots of trees, flowers and it was well kept. Check mark. We were greeted by staff members who were quite friendly yet professional. Check mark.

Our tour began. As we sat in a room listening to all the wonderful things this home offered, I was distracted by some grunting noises in the hall. A woman in a wheelchair was looking at us. I smiled at her and tried to refocus.

The intake worker spoke to Dawn and me. I was not dismissed as having no value to add to the conversation. Check mark.

I communicated the importance of living a life of dignity and embracing each day. She agreed. Check mark.

We began to look at the different kinds of rooms which are available. Depending on what you can afford, there are single, double and four people rooms. There is a large difference in each kind of room. Hmm. I did not know how to evaluate my choices. This tour was becoming harder to understand and decide. No check mark and no x. I would have to come back to this and mull over the possibilities.

We turned into another hallway. Immediately, my eyes stung, and I was overcome with the smell of urine. I stopped. I interrupted our tour guide. "To be blunt, this smells like urine." I informed her. She seemed surprised. She paused for a moment and then said, it depends on the time of the day. I'm not sure what that meant, nor did I really care. Her talking began to fade away in the distance as I continued to take in the horrible smell. This is terrible, I thought. More than one person causes this. For me to smell it in the hallway, means there is a lot of urine. I was horrified. It depends on the time of day. Really? What does the time of day have to do with anything? How can a person live with dignity in this stench? I would NEVER live here. What happened to the comment about dignity?

I stopped listening to our tour guide. I went through the rest of the building so I could compare it to others. As we walked down another hallway, the lady in the wheelchair, who I saw earlier, pointed at me. She motioned for me to come to her. I did and put my hand on hers and smiled. She took my hand and brought it to her dry mouth and softly kissed my hand. I looked into her eyes and told her thank you. I had a desire to sit down beside her and talk with her. Instead, she gave me another soft kiss. It was then time for me to go.

I was told that she never does that. I wonder why I was singled out. When she looked into my eyes, did she now how sad I was? Did my tears, that were starting to build, give me away? Did she have a room in the urine stench hallway? I can only wonder.

As I closed the building door behind me, I thought to myself, I will never be back here again. But unfortunately, the smell of urine in that hallway, will never leave me. On to the next long-term care facility.

What a Wonderful World

Date: June 10th, 2013

I have insomnia. I was sleeping for a bit, but then woke up. As I lay in bed, I began to think about the day I had. I know I must write about two extraordinary events.

To set the tone of the day, I need you for you to think of Louis Armstrong's song, "What a wonderful world."

Today, I was busy in the yard. Weeds seem to come in some new classification of "weeds-on-steroids." There was much delight in yanking them out so my flowers could show off their true beauty. Shiloh, my big brown lab was out with me enjoying the sun. It was a good day.

I was focused on removing some of these weeds-on-steroids, when suddenly I heard this high-pitched, squeaky sound. Quickly turning around, I saw Shiloh nosing in the grass some tiny creature. I grabbed his collar and brought him into the house. I examined the area and to my surprise discovered a tiny bunny. It was pink with a bit of black, perhaps 2 inches long, with its eyes tightly shut. Wow! Looking around, I found an indent in the long grass. A tiny nest with another baby bunny was nestled into its warm surroundings. Not wanting to touch it, I used two sticks to gently move the bunny back into its home. I then covered it back up with grass and white fur fluffs. Extraordinary! Never in my life have I seen such a thing. And here one was in my own back yard, hiding in plain view. Excited by my findings, I went into the house to share the news with Dawn. Her eyes lite up as well.

I wanted to know more about these little babies, so my quick googling found a few facts for me:

✓ rabbits won't reject their offspring if you touch them
✓ a female rabbit will only nurse her litter a few minutes once or twice at night
✓ the rabbit doe (mother) will be out of the nest most of the time, and
✓ the doe pulls out some of its own fur to line the nest.

Humming to myself "what a wonderful world" I continued my work. Suddenly, a quick motion caught my eye. Right in front of me, a hummingbird danced about the flowers, extracting nectar as it went. Its shiny green metallic back shone in the sunlight. I watched it in awe; it seemed unaware of me. As quickly as it came, it left. Extraordinary.

Within one hour of each other, I saw two extraordinary events that I have never witnessed before. All within my own backyard. It made me pause and wonder. Do I have extra sensor since having Frontotemporal Lobe Dementia (FTD)? Perhaps I am looking at the world differently and therefore, seeing things I never saw before. Perhaps I am more in tune with my surroundings?

I do not know the answers to the questions I ask myself. What I do know is today, I saw two extraordinary events and I live in a wonderful world.

The Changing of the Gardener

Date: June 17th, 2013

I come from a line of proud Scottish gardeners. I am told that my Great Grandfather was an estate gardener at Ardclach, Nainshire, Scotland in 1902.

As far back as my memories take me, I can always remember my parents working the soil producing beautiful flowers and vegetables. My father always tried to grow roses with varied success. He liked to present my Mom with a rose showing his love for her. How sweet is that?

My parents have not put in a garden for the last few years. Although, they did have a few plants on their balcony. Just enough to get their hands dirty; and have something to show-off and talk about. When they downsized, I had the good fortune to obtain my fathers long gardening shovel. I don't know how old it is, but it was his favourite. It has moved a lot of earth in its time!

This year, our garden was on the late side of being put in. Dawn asked if I was going to do it this year. I responded with an "of course" because I am not able to imagine a springtime without one. As she prodded me gently to get moving on it, I realized that things have changed. This year, I found it overwhelming. I needed help with turning the ground, buying the plants, seeding, etc.

As I contemplated this, I knew the time had come for the handing off the shovel to the next generation – Brianna. If you speak to a carer of someone with Frontotemporal Lobe Dementia (FTD), they will tell you that it is common for the person to eventually be unable to plant and take care of the garden. It is, as they say, "the new norm."

If you think about it, there are many steps to gardening. It can be overwhelming, without the person realizing the issue. It is not always easy to articulate.

For someone to live well with dementia, a helping hand can go along way in being successful. With Brianna's help, we were able to turn the earth, pick out our plants, plant, fertilize and we are now waiting impatiently for them to start producing.

Brianna has picked this season first batch of rhubarb and has made her first pot of stewed rhubarb. It has already been given to Grandma and Grandpa Wighton for a treat. It made them proud.

We have begun making plans on how in the Fall, we will use our tomatoes and make jars of salsa. We have never done this before, so it will be an adventure.

And my Dad's long shovel – has been ceremoniously been given to Brianna. It is my hope that she too will teach her children about flowers and gardens. When she is older, she will reflect on the days we spent in the garden, laughing, and enjoying our time together.

As is the changing of the guard, the changing of the gardener has begun. I know Brianna will always help me in making sure my hands get a little dirty each Spring. Together, we will enjoy the fruits of our labour and bury dementia for as long as we can.

Care – What Helps, What Hurts?

Date: July 2nd, 2013

Last week, the Waterloo Wellington Dementia Network hosted a successful one-day educational event for professional care partners. The focus was the importance of developing good rapport and caring relationships with those that the health professional supports persons with dementia.

Two speakers of the event included Mr. Bob Kallonen, Chief Operating Officer of Schlegel Villages, and Dr. Elaine Weirsma, PhD, Associate Professor, Department of Health Sciences, and Advisor, Interdisciplinary Certificate in Dementia Studies, Lakehead University. Their goal was to challenge the approximately 110 participants to enhance relationships between all carers.

In the middle of these two engaging speakers, a panel of four additional speakers shared with the audience their personal experiences of professional relationships and dementia. Dawn and I had the wonderful opportunity to be a part of this panel. We had the pleasure of joining Brenda Hounam, Person with Dementia, and Anne Hopewell, Carer for a Person with Dementia – her husband Ron.

Brenda, advocate extraordinaire, started our panel discussion by sharing some of her personal experiences of various medical relationships. Brenda has a wealth of knowledge as she has been diagnosed with early onset Alzheimer's several years ago. Anne, then took over and shared some stories with tips on enhancing relationships.

Next, it was me. I couldn't wait to get a hold of that microphone! This was my moment. The last few days, I had worked hard at trying to capture my thoughts on paper. The reality of it is, I have

experienced numerous negative conversations with some members of the medical community. It is hard to forget. The important thing for me to remember was that the attendees are the individuals who *wanted* to learn how to enhance their own relationships with their patients. Therefore, it was crucial I communicated points which someone could easily and readily implement during the next meeting with someone with dementia.

I had boiled down my experiences to the following "take-aways":

1. Be aware of the power the medical community wields during documentation of reports and the potential negative impact it may have on the patient's financial insurance and ultimately wellbeing.

2. Question yourself about your own stereotypes. When you are working with someone who has dementia, ask yourself if you are comparing their symptoms to someone who is late stage Alzheimer's. It is shocking how often this happens.

It was then Dawn's turn to convince this audience of utilizing some of her suggestions to enhance relationships. People were busy taking notes as she shared the following:

✓ Use email to provide updates to the professionals. Ultimately, this becomes a journal of sorts, and enables people to review the case from the beginning.

✓ Avoid possible anxiousness and agitation of the patient, by reducing appointment wait times. Have the carer call ahead to confirm the appointment is on time. If not, let them alter it accordingly.

✓ Be careful of the language you use. Be empathetic.

✓ Be the barrier of bad news. Instead of having the carer communicate things like revoking a licence, do it for them. It is much easier if the bad news comes directly from the medical community; and

✓ Prior to a diagnosis, know what the disease entails. If you do not, do the necessary research.

Perhaps the best way to summarize the object of the panel is by a quote from advocate, Kate Swaffer, (Advocate and activist for aged and dementia care) "I think for some people they forget 'the human feeling person behind the illness/symptoms' and thus they forget to approach each interaction with the care that any relationship deserves."

I come from a training background. Therefore, I'm very interested in if our words will change any behaviours of members of the audience. In other words, how do you measure success of the panel? For me, if I can help even just one person, then I have succeeded.

I'm happy to report we have succeeded. After the event, I received an email from one of the participants. She stated: I was at the Dementia Network Conference and your experience has left a true impression on me. We can do things better; I know we can, and I want to do as much as possible to get your voice out into Primary Care.

We will be meeting with this individual in a few weeks to discuss our experiences to increase awareness. The Alzheimer Society of Ontario has been given funding to work on a campaign that will strengthen linkages with many groups to better serve people with dementia and their caregivers. I'm looking forward to being a part of this project to enhance carer relationships. Well-done!

The Search Continues

Date: July 7th, 2013

This past May, Dawn and I began our search for finding three possible long-term care facilities for me.

To remind you, it is our hope that I will always remain at home, so this is putting a "plan b" together – just in case.

It is discouraging in that I have yet to hear of anyone who has later stage Frontotemporal Lobe Dementia (FTD), live at home until the end. bvFTD, the kind I have, it is exceedingly difficult for the carer to manage the challenging symptoms and possible aggressiveness.

CCAC is waiting for me to return the paperwork listing up to three facilities. Due to some facilities that have up to a five-year waiting list, it is important I submit my paperwork in a timely fashion. That basically means – now.

As we drove to my second long-term care facility, I tried to be positive. The first facility we toured had an incredible urine stench in its one hallway. I tried to push that memory way back in my brain. I know they can't all be like that.

I could feel myself getting anxious as we drove up to a small, modern looking building. I took a few minutes to glance over the exterior of the building. It seemed nice enough – some well-kept gardens surrounded the building. Check mark.

I took a deep breath and entered the building. The entrance had several people in wheelchairs sitting in the hallway. Some people were asleep, while others just sat there motionless. It threw me off. I wondered why they were there.

There was a small front desk, but nobody was there to help us. Hmm. Dawn stopped a nurse and told her we had an appointment to be shown the facility. The nurse quickly determined the individual we were to see was not yet at work. She checked the schedule and he was scheduled to be there. She called him at home and was told he was still at home but would be there soon. She added his home was just down the street so it wouldn't take him long. Hmm.

At this point, I asked if someone else was available and was told that the other two people who could do that also were not at work currently.

The nurse brought us down to a nice room which had a fireplace, some good comfy chairs, puzzle boards, and pictures of past residents. I wondered why the people sitting in the hallway were not in this room. It was just Dawn and I and one other resident. We waited. The room's quietness soon became deafening to me. I started to get agitated and restless. We waited some more.

I could not understand why the individual was not even at work. We had a 11:00 appointment confirmed. We did not receive a telephone call saying he would be late. Thoughts ran through my head. Is this the way this facility is run - show up at work anytime you want? It is O. K. to make people wait for you, even when you have an appointment? How does this lack of professionalism and lack of respect translate into taking excellent care of the residents? Hmm.

We had enough. We retreated the way we came in and stopped the same nurse. She looked embarrassed and apologized for her manager not being there. From the way she looked, I had a feeling this was not the first time this manager had been late for an appointment. We told her it was not her fault. We asked her to inform her manager of our disappointment and we would not be back.

As we headed back to our car, I noticed a man heading into the front entrance. I asked him his name. Sure enough, he was the person who was supposed to show us the facility 25 minutes ago. To my surprise, he did not apologize and told us he had a personal delivery at his home. He added that he could now show us the facility. I told him that I was not interested. He obviously did not respect us or our time. He failed to take any accountability and seemed surprised that I was upset. He obviously was not getting it. He asked me why I would be nervous to see the facility. Dawn came to my aid and reminded him of the lengthy conversion they had a few days ago. Not only was he late, but he obviously had not reviewed his notes stating that a woman of 46 years old was looking for a residence for herself. As he stood there looking at us with his mouth open, we drove away.

I don't understand it. For anyone to view a long-term care facility is nerve racking. Especially, if it is you who is the possible resident. There are so many thoughts flying around in your brain. You are anxious and nervous. To be met with such incredulous disrespect is frankly disheartening.

The search continues.

Please Sir – May I Have More Sugar?

Date: July 13th, 2013

When you have Frontotemporal Lobe Dementia (FTD) like me, you can expect to experience different symptoms. Some symptoms never leave, and others may go as quickly as they come. Some examples of symptoms which I have experienced/experiencing are:

➤ Impulsive

➤ Poor judgement

➤ Withdraw of interest in activities

➤ Easily distracted

➤ Lack of attention to personal hygiene

➤ Drinking to excess

➤ Abrupt mood changes

➤ Lack of empathy

➤Impatience and aggression

➤ Trouble finding the right word

➤ Memory loss

➤ Muscle spasms

➤ Swallowing problems

In addition to the list above, there is another two common symptoms I have been experiencing for about the last six months:
food fad 1 – eating excessive amounts of sugar food, and
food fad 2 – wanting to eat only breakfast cereal in addition to sugar.

Before we get too much further, let me give you some background on my normal eating habits. Basically, I am a meat and potato type of girl. I enjoy eating various types of ethnic food. But I have never been known to lick my plate clean if there are salads on it. Greens are OK. If I feel like I'm in need of them.

Food fad 1 – sugar, started innocently enough with a desire to eat some sour keys bought in small bags. At first, I would eat a few at a time. But quickly, it became large handfuls to ultimately eating the entire bag in one sitting. If you have ever eaten a sour key candy you would know that it contains a large amount of sugar on just one candy. Imagine, eating the entire bag!

This is when my "split personality" emerged. The "Good Person" would tell myself that this is very unhealthy; I should not be eating these large quantities of candies. It tried to reason with the "Bad Person" pleading to consume less sugar. In the beginning, Good Person won many of the battles. I would wrap up the candies and put them away for another day. Or, I would only eat one colour, like red, and then put the bag away.

As time went by, Good Person started to lose more of the battles. Not only would I eat an entire bag of candies, but I would look for more to eat. This is all in one sitting! Dawn tried different methods to reduce my sugar intake. She didn't buy all the candy. When she did buy some, she hid the bags and gave me a little baggy with just a few assorted treats. Some days this would work and others...not so much. She tried to encourage me to eat more fruit and other food containing natural sugar. I resisted. While she was at work, I would hunt down the bags secured in their hiding spots. If I found them, I would hold the bags in triumph and the feast would begin.

I also had another trick to get my sugar high. I would go into the store to pick up something and buy chocolate or candy. I would then hide them in my coat and put them secretly away at home. I believe this is where I can use the word hoarding!

A few weeks ago, I switched from sour keys and soft sugar candy to toffee. I LOVE toffee. While we were grocery shopping, I picked out a bag of assorted types of toffee. To Dawn's horror, the entire bag was gone by the next day. We tried one more bag. It too was demolished in record breaking time.

Good Person tried to slow things down by having me eat only certain flavours at a time. First it was all green, then red, then blue, etc. I ate the entire bag in two days. This is when I knew Bad Person had truly won out the battle of sugar. I did not feel guilty about doing this. I didn't feel sick from all the sugar. It seemed that I could not open any type of candy without eating the entire contents.

While Good Person and Bad Person battled over my sugar intake, another food fad began. It started innocently enough. Instead of eating one bowl of cereal in the morning, I began to eat two bowls.

Eventually, I began to eat cereal for lunch. And yes, you guessed it, I started wanting only cereal for dinner. We tried various strategies to overcome this fad. First, we always made sure I was eating healthy cereal. It was odd, but I didn't crave sugary cereal. I liked the ones with granola in it. Our cupboards were full of cereal boxes. Dawn tried all different kinds of foods to lure me back to eating properly. Many a time she would hear, "I don't like that." She would shake her head in disbelief as I was saying that to foods, I used to enjoy eating.

All this gluttonous eating has caused large weight gains. I have already gained a lot because of some of my medication. This now puts me about 35 lbs higher than my normal weight. Over the last two weeks, my insatiable desire to eat sugar has dissipated. Finally, I can eat fruit and it will take care of that craving.

Also, my interest in food has somewhat come back. However, there are still many foods which do not look appetizing and I refuse to eat them. But, its much better than it was. Oral stimulation is very much a common symptom with people having FTD. This also can include putting objects in one's mouth.

With all symptoms we can only do our best with them. For now, at least I won't be asking for more sugar – please.

Shiloh – A Woman's Best Friend

Date: July 17th, 2013

For most of my life, I have been a "cat person." I have had many beautiful cats that have entertained me with their personalities. My all-time favourite was a Main Coon named "Jack." Jack the Cat was rescued by my friend Marie. He was in terrible shape due from being out in the cold winter, lack of food, water and warmth. After a visit to the vet, Marie and Theresa brought him to my home. When he was let out of his cat carrier, I almost fell over looking at the sight of the ugliest cat I had ever seen. The vet had to shave him right down because of his matted fur. We laughed at this craziest looking cat. Another friend, Linda, coined the name: Jack. This is a short form for the cat "hitting the jackpot" on living with me. Eventually, he turned into a beautiful big boy of 20lbs.

But I have digressed. On our fourth Valentines day celebration, Dawn stated she wanted a Labrador dog for a present for me. He would join our already formed pack of 2 other dogs – Leo and Riley. It took a lot of convincing for me to concede and agree.

Dawn did a lot of research into local breeders and eventually discovered one who she liked. This breeder was scheduled to visit with his three brown labs. One was the mother, and the other two were the pups. This is when our family was introduced to Shiloh. He was the calmer dog of the two pups being shown to us. He was the perfect pup with big paws and ran with his butt almost running faster than the front part of his body.

Although Shiloh was the biggest of our dogs, he always was the calmer and best dispositioned. He even let our cat sleep in his bed or drink his water. Everyone loves Shiloh.

This past year, Shiloh became the only one left in our pack of dogs. I found having three dogs too stimulating and I became agitated. We made the extremely hard decision to adopt Leo and Riley out to a good home. We all miss them but know its for the best.

Its curious, as the longer I am sick with Frontotemporal Lobe Dementia (FTD), the more Shiloh seems to bond with me. If he is not lying in his bed, usually he will be laying at my feet. If I go outside without him, he has been known to sit at the door whining until I return. Shiloh and I are thick as thieves. I whisper my secrets to him and tell him of my frustrations and triumphs. He is such a wonderful listener and never interrupts me.

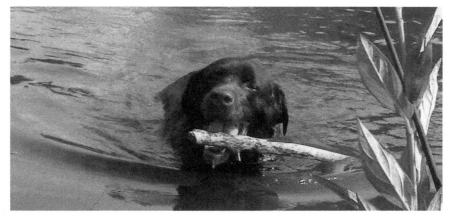

Shiloh

An important thing that he does is he calms me down. If I am feeling anxious, sad, or agitated, just by patting him I begin to feel better. He is incredibly good for my emotional well-being.

Before my diagnosis, I was researching into the St. John Ambulance Therapy Dog Program. I believed Shiloh would make a perfect candidate. These dogs can be found in hospitals, retirement residents, and long-term care facilities. From visiting with a dog, patients talk more, participate in activities, eat, and sleep better. Overall, their quality of life improves.

Once I was diagnosed with FTD, Shiloh has become my own therapy dog. He is wonderful for me. Therefore, I found it as no surprise when, today, I read about two specially trained dogs in the UK, becoming the first dogs to assist in helping people with early-stage dementia. The dogs, responding to sound alerts, can help with regular hydration, medication, and toilet use. In addition, they can also be trained to provide orientation when outside of the home.

Just like me with my Shiloh, the social and emotional benefits are huge for the two individuals who have received a dementia dog. From my own experiences as a person with dementia, I can attest to the therapeutic effect a dog has on my mood.

There is a reason why dogs are called "man's best friend." They are loyal, comforting and look past any physical or emotional challenges someone may have.

I look forward to watching the Dementia Dog program become internationally known and helping those with dementia. I believe this will happen relatively quickly as its website is receiving so many visitors, that it has exceeded its internet bandwidth limit. Awesome job team!

Happy Birthday

Date: August 4th, 2013

It was 41 years ago today, when my Dawnie Girl was born. I am so grateful to her parents for their gift to the world.

Dawn and I met about 11.5 years ago. Since that time, we have become inseparable. It was a whirlwind romance and we both knew that we had found "the one." Included in this package was Brianna who was seven years old. Two for the price of one!

The first birthday we celebrated together was when she turned 30 years old. I hosted a barbecue for family and friends in the trailer park where we were staying. It was a great success as this gang toasted to Dawn. It was then I began to see how loved she was by the people who knew her.

On reflection, I don't remember most of her birthday celebrations. Although, I do remember one of my gifts which was a wonderful surprise for her. On her big day, she woke up with travel bags beside her. With a coffee in her hand, I escorted her to the car for me to transport her to a surprise destination. Off we went to Niagara-on-the-Lake to experience the wonderful gifts this area has to offer. It was a magical few days of enjoying each others company.

Birthdays are especially important to Dawn. They are the one day of the year in which it is all about the birthday person. It is not about the gifts, but rather the simple things like coffee served in bed, phone calls from old friends and family, cards in the mail, and birthday cake.

One of the symptoms of Frontotemporal Dementia, is that it becomes more difficult to make decisions, and organize events. We saw that quite clearly this year as I did not organize anything and had to rely on Dawn telling me what she would like for a present. Brianna then went out and picked up the surprises. Dawn, understanding me and my forgetfulness, gently reminded me to buy a cake. It is our tradition to always have a birthday cake. I am grateful to her for sure enough I had forgotten.

Yesterday, began the early celebration. My nephew, Jeremy, and his three kids stayed with us for a night. The kids had made wonderful bird houses for Dawn. My brother Mark and Mary Anne helped with the celebration by bringing over a plate of brownies with a birthday candle in the middle. She received two bouquets of flowers and a small birthday cake from someone we barely know.

Today, is Dawn's day. Brianna and I will do our best to pamper her and make sure she knows how much we love her. I am so fortunate and blessed to have Dawn in my life. I couldn't imagine it without her.

Happy Birthday my Dawnie Girl – I love you.

The Cottage

Date: August 7th, 2013

A few days ago, My Girls and I packed up the car, jumped in and headed off for an adventure. We love adventures, and this was one we had been looking forward to for several weeks. Our destination was Miller Lake located up in the beautiful Bruce Peninsula. My friend, Sue, has a family cottage right on the lake. We planned on staying up for two nights with her and her husband Pete.

Sue and I have been friends since grade six. That means 34 years. It's an easy friendship where at times we can go for a long period of time without chatting with each other. Just recently, we have rekindled our relationship and have picked up where we left off. Our relationship goes back to a time of childhood – prior to our significant others and children. It was a carefree time of riding bikes, playing endless card games, fishing, and swimming. As we grew up, our lives naturally changed as we met our soul mates, became parents, and followed our careers.

A few months ago, Sue reached out to me as she had heard I have been diagnosed with Frontotemporal Dementia (FTD). Sometimes, it can be unnerving to reach out to someone who has dementia and is newly diagnosed. You do not always know what to expect or say. Sue was unfazed and was open to education. That's a true friend.

During our last visit, we scheduled a time to visit Sue and Pete at the cottage. A few days ago, we arrived at Miller Lake. It had been over 30 years since I was last there. As Dawn pulled into the driveway, I immediately recognized the cottage and was brought back to be a little girl. I could see Sue and I running for the cottage door and opening it up to begin our adventures at the cottage.

Recently, I was asked what ways my memory is affected, long and short-term. During our visit with Sue and Pete, it was evident to all how intact my long-term memory is. Short-term memory... not so much.

I easily recalled those days so long ago. I remember the chopping of wood, pumping water, names of roads, the fruitless efforts of many fishing trips, furniture, and Sue making a turkey. In comparison, while updating her contact list, Sue confirmed with me my address.

Although I haven't been there for five years, I acknowledged it was a correct current address. Dawn helped in supplying the proper one.

During our stay, the weather was very cool, and the wind was strong. It was not good boating weather as white caps crashed against the beach. But that didn't matter. We enjoyed lounging by the fire, napping and of course eating. Shiloh and I spent some wonderful time on the dock just taking in the beauty of Miller Lake. He also had quite a workout swimming against the waves as he retrieved the stick I had thrown.

The highlight of our holiday occurred on our second evening. The weather had calmed down and the lake became still. Brianna and Pete decided it was a good time to fish and off they went to troll the waters. Two hours later, they came back into the cottage in great spirits. Both had caught a large fish with pictures to prove it. For the next bit, the energy in the cottage was charged as we heard the retelling of their fish tales. !

Earlier that day, Brianna had commented to me how wonderful it was to be in a place I enjoyed as a child. It was something that she treasured me sharing with her. For a few days, Brianna and Dawn had a taste of my carefree childhood days. They relished in it and it acted like a salve helping to repair any open wounds.

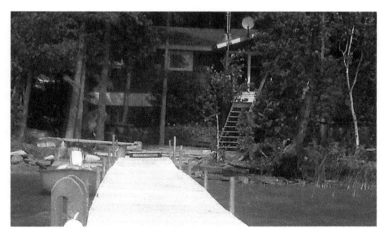

The Cottage

I am reminded of "silver and gold friends." Sue and Peter are gold nuggets. They have assisted me and my family to live with dignity and embrace the day. I know they will be there to help us charter through life's choppy waters and find a peaceful area for us to sail through our journey of life once again.

It Takes a Village...

Date: August 25th, 2013

One of the first poems I learned was "Casey at the Bat" by Ernest Lawrence Thayer. It is my favourite poem telling of the story of the crowd hero, Casey, of the Mudville town baseball team. You are kept on the edge of your seat, stanza after stanza, until the final sentence of the poem when you learn the outcome of his turn at bat.

Yesterday, much like the crowd described in this poem, I was on the edge of my seat, watching our niece, Brontae, play baseball in the championship game at a local tournament. It was an even match of experience and ability. Depending on which side you were on, cries of "nooo..." echoed the umpires "striiiike!"

When Brontae's turn came to bat, it seemed that the crowd was extra loud in encouraging her. The reason for that is simple – there was a large contingent of family members watching her. Besides Dawn and I, other family spectators included: Grandmas Joyce and Helen, Aunt Deion and Uncle Dan, Aunt Wendy, Coby a family friend, Dylan – her brother, and her Mom and Dad (who also is the coach).

As she confidently strode towards the plate, my mind wandered. I took a quick look around at this collection of family members. Each person was quite different. Unique individuals have been created from past experiences, triumphs, disappointments, and heartaches. Yet, we all had one common goal which was to support Brontae who we all love.

This made me think of the African proverb, "It takes a whole village to raise a child." Each one of us, regardless of age, sex, and background, has something to teach Brontae. We have a shared vision, values, and collective responsibility to help properly raise her and support her parents.

Although being diagnosed with dementia, it is still my responsibility to contribute in the shared responsibility of raising this special young lady. It is important for me to think of others and their needs and not just my own. It is my hope that as time passes, I will impart to Brontae my motto of carpe diem: seize the day and place no trust in tomorrow.

Brontae does not just interact with her parents. She is a social person who has many interactions with many different individuals. Collectively, we can be thought of as the village.

My mind shifted back to the game when Brontae was at the plate with bat raised. Although I have dementia, it felt great to be part of the village cheering for her. Just like my cheers, my love is no different from someone else. Unlike my favourite poem, the mighty Casey who struck out – our hero – Brontae, brought joy to the town of Southampton. She hit the ball and raced to the base to be declared "safeeeee!"

Project Lifesaver

Date: August 30th, 2013

I have had a heavy heart for the last 10 days. It was then that George Handzik, an 84-year-old man with dementia, was identified as missing. He was last seen at 4:30 August 20th, riding his bicycle. He was reported missing to police at 7:30 p.m. that same day. He is still missing.

I have tried to imagine being Mr. Handzik; Placing myself in an imaginary setting of being lost and not knowing what to do or where to go. Perhaps I am hurt, and I am unable to get to a place where I can be helped. I try to imagine how frighten I would be. The problem is – I just can't. I have been lost before. I felt an immediate response of being scared to the situations. But it was a quick feeling as I got my bearings in a short period of time.

I have also tried to imagine being Mr. Handzik's carer or a member of his family. Again, this is outside something I can imagine. It is too disturbing.

Nearly 200,000 Ontarians have dementia. Fifty percent of those who go missing for 24 hours become seriously injured or die. Anyone with dementia can go missing with no warning signs. Having Frontotemporal Lobe Dementia (FTD), means I am part of that statistic. And because of that statistic, my partner, Dawn, and I have discussed the possibility of me wandering. To help ease some of this concern, always I wear a MedicAlert® bracelet and am registered with the program of Safely Home®. It is for people with dementia to be easily identified in case we become lost. This is a wonderful program and I strongly encourage people to use it. However, in the case of Mr. Handzik, even if he is wearing a Safely Home® bracelet, unfortunately, it will still not help him as he must be found for it to be beneficial.

There is another program called Project Lifesaver, which is supported by local police services in some Ontario communities, that would be beneficial in a situation like this one. Participants wear a bracelet that is a battery-operated transmitter. It emits a unique radio frequency every second, 24 hours a day. This transmitter has the proven ability to transmit through obstacles, concrete, buildings, and heavy forest. When a carer notifies their local police that someone has gone missing, specially trained police officers search for the missing person.

Project Lifesaver is an international program which boasts that most who wander are found within a few miles from home, and search times have been reduced from hours and days to minutes. It's recovery time is an average of 30 minutes.

The website of York Regional Police does a good job at explaining more about this program and you can download an application form. This non-profit program costs $300 for the bracelet and an additional monthly cost of $10 for the replacement of battery and bracelet when needed.

It is a terrible, rainy evening. My heart is still heavy in concern for Mr. Handzik. I pray that he is quickly found and is brought back to his loved ones.

Time to Examine My Personal Motto

Date: September 8th, 2013

It was one year ago, on September 5th, that my life changed forever. It was on that day I was diagnosed with Frontotemporal Lobe Dementia (FTD).

I suppose you can call it a one-year anniversary. But I associate anniversaries with parties and champagne. I partook in neither. What I have done is a lot of reflection on this past year. It is a bit strange as it seems longer than a year. I think that perhaps the lengthy time it took to be diagnosed with FTD feeds into this timeline. At minimum, that tacks on another four years.

As many people will tell you who are diagnosed after a long struggle, it was a relief. I finally have something to call this "thing." It now gives me the ability to put a plan together and adjust my life accordingly. I now know the kind of help me and my family need. I can now refer in concrete terms (as much as that means) to symptoms, medications, tests, and future.

I have always been a person who does not like too much grey. I prefer black and white. It provides sound boundaries that I know I am to operate in, little room for confusion or error. Having dementia means that I now live in the grey. Boundaries can change quickly and easily. I have tried to learn to adopt to these changes. It has been quite the learning curve.

It wasn't long after my diagnosis, that I was introduced to and adopted for my personal motto: carpe diem. In loose translation, this Latin phrase means "seize the day;" be spontaneous; just go for it. I have not kept this motto to myself but rather have shared it with anyone who will listen to me. I have publicly spoken and written about carp diem.

While I was in the corporate world, at the key milestones and at the end of projects, the team took the time to evaluate our effort. We would compare our results to the intended objectives and determine our success. We would challenge ourselves on how we could improve so future projects would benefit from our learning of the previous project. I found this to be an excellent methodology for project management.

I consider my life not as a project but as a journey. However, I feel I can still use this methodology of evaluating how successful I feel I am in my life.

With that said, I bring you back to one year ago when my goal was to live carpe diem. I now am at a milestone point, where I am reflecting on if this has been successful. Remembering the definition of carpe diem, I am quite happy to state I believe I have been very successful.

I changed when I was diagnosed. I decided to be an advocate for those with dementia. I want to help dispel stigma and educate all those who will listen. I want to be proactive in obtaining support and putting my "ducks-in-a-row." I want to step into the limelight and stand up to speak for those who are unable. I want to share my journey by writing journals and promoting them. But more importantly than all of that, I want to be a better spouse, mother, daughter, sister, aunt, and friend. I have searched and found a deeper relationship with God. I have renewed relationships and enjoyed meeting new people and making new friends.

Carpe diem is not just my personal motto, it has become my families. We try not to take things for granted anymore. We work hard to try and speak more gently with each other and be more encouraging. We have done a wonderful job at making new memories and jumping at chances for adventures. We are more apt to try new foods and restaurants. And each day, we tell each other of our love for them.

So, when I compare what carpe diem means to how I have lived my life this past year, I must say it has been a wonderful success. But this is success as a team. Dawn and Brianna have had a stellar performance.

Support has come from all different avenues that have helped me in achieving living for the day.

I have yet to define goals for myself for this coming year. For the new few days, I think I am just going to enjoy the wonderful feeling of all the successes.

Thank you to each one of you who have helped me live with dignity and carpe diem.

Pioneers

Date: September 18th, 2013

Michael James McCoy is my great-great grandfather. He was born in Ireland in 1828 and died in Moore Township, Ontario in 1907 at the age of 78. What is interesting about him, is that on his death certificate it states cause of death as "Senile Decay" and the length of illness as "2 months."

It is in the same year, 1907, that Alzheimer's disease (AD) was first recognized and named by Alois Alzheimer. However, it wasn't until the 1970's before it was considered a major disease. And in 1978 the Alzheimer Society Canada was formed.

Today, I was at a monthly meeting where I am a member of a team working on a self-management project. It is led by a MAREP representative and hosted by my local Alzheimer Society. Members of the team consists of people with dementia, carers, MAREP representatives as well as a member from the Alzheimer Society.

One of the major topics of discussion was communication with family and friends. This sparked a great deal of conversation with everyone contributing and offering their viewpoint. As I listened to the comments and stories, it dawned on me how fortunate I am. Members of this project team are working hard to help develop an educational package to be used by those with dementia. Not only that, but the project team itself has representatives from the population it is trying to support.

Beside me sat Brenda Hounam, advocate extraordinaire. Recently, she shared with me a bit of history of what things were like when she was first diagnosed in the year 2000 at the age of 53. People with dementia did not go to conferences and speak; they did not attend support groups; you would not find them at meetings that discussed plans and projects to help those with dementia; they simply were talked about and not talked to or asked to be involved.

In fact, Brenda attended her first meeting pretending to be a carer and not someone with dementia. It was with the encouragement of a member of the Alzheimer Society that she began to stand-up and talk to people about having dementia. In this area of the world, this was a first. People just didn't do that. Through Brenda and some other pioneers, the philosophy of By Us for Us emerged. It is a wonderful and strong philosophy that I will adopt for a new e-newsletter project I will be starting.

We have come along way since the year 2000. But before we get patting on our back too much, there is still much work to be completed. This year I was on a panel at a conference for professionals who help people with dementia. Shockingly, it was the first time the organizers had people with dementia speaking. I'm happy to say it was a success.

Today, sitting beside Brenda, it made me think that I too am a pioneer, albeit second generation. In 1861, my great-great grandfather owned 100 acres in Moore Township. He travelled from Ireland across the ocean landing on Wolfe Island. He travelled south settling in this area. He than began the arduous task of clearing the land and building a home. In this year, 80 acres were still woods. I admire him and his tenacity.

Like him, I too have a lot of work to do on the lay of the land. It requires a good deal of tilling before it will be able to fully produce the fruits of our labour.

I imagine my great-great grandfather being excited when he started off on his voyage crossing the ocean so many years ago. He must have dreamt about the life he was going to have. Through his hard work, he will help in making a brighter future for his family for generations to come. His vision came true.

I am excited, as well, thinking about all the possibilities that is in front of us. It is my plan to work as hard as I can to help other pioneers improve life for those with dementia.

The Road Not Taken

September 30th, 2013

For you Robert Frost fans, you will have immediately recognized "The Road Not Taken" as the title of his famous poem published in 1916. Recently, a dear old friend mailed a copy of it to me. I have reread it numerous times contemplating the intended meaning by the poet. I have concluded it is more important for me to develop my own interpretation than depending on others.

To remind you of his words, here is a summary: The speaker is walking in the woods and comes to a fork in the road. He stands for some time contemplating which road to take. Both look the same, covered with some fallen leaves. Neither looks trodden on. He chooses one of the roads realizing that he will not be back to also take the other road. Much later in life, the speaker wonders about the other road he did not choose but sighs with contentment with the one he did.

I'm sure you can appreciate the symbolism in this poem – having to choose a path in life with sometimes little to guide us in our decision. When reflecting on this choice, we can sometimes get caught in the "what if I had chosen the other path..."

As I reread Frosts' poem reflecting on my own symbolic forks in the road, I realize that I have had a few key turns in life. And here I am today. Someone suggested to me, that we do not pick our own path, but rather it picks us. That has given me great thought.

Tomorrow, I will begin another adventure with MAREP. We will begin to tape a new web video series titled "Living Well with Dementia." This series is about me (the host who is newly diagnosed with dementia) who will take a journey each episode and meet others who have dementia. From these positive individuals, I will learn from their experiences. From the road each has journeyed, they will share with me their personal experiences on how to live a meaningful and full life with dementia.

I would hazard a guess that during the filming this week, each person will be reflecting on their own "The Road Not Taken." Once again, I feel fortunate and blessed to be in the unique position of learning from others who have gone before me on the road called Dementia.

With the help of these individual's insight, shared lessons learned, and positive energy – I believe the road I will travel will be easier than the traveller before me. As far as the road choosing me... I think there may be some merit in that.

Tomorrow, Dawn, Brianna and I will discuss in front of video camera's my journey into dementia, as well as the future of education and support. Whether the road chooses me, or I choose the road, what is essential is I live well with dementia. Only time will tell.

First Game – First Concussion

Date: October 2nd, 2013

When I woke up this morning and turned on the TV., Canadian news was flooded by clips of last nights fight between Montreal Canadians enforcer George Parros with Toronto Maple Leafs Colton Orr. The cheering crowd turned deathly silent when Parros, with his helmet still on, while fighting tripped face first to the ice. He did not move. Orr quickly signalled for a medical team to assist. Parros was carted off and is now being treated in the hospital for a concussion.

Being Canadian, I have the love for hockey weaved into my very core. I do not watch all the games but like to tune in when the playoffs begin. I then find my seat on the couch with a beer in one hand and chips in the other. For me, a "good game" consists of excellent passing, checking and awesome goal tending. It does not consist of dirty hits, and enforcers nailing other players. It does not consist of fights.

A good friend of mine is a NHL Linesman. He's being doing this job for several years. I remember incredibly early in his career; he was chastised by his manager as he did not let two players fight "long enough." He jumped in too quickly to stop the fight. For that, he received a verbal warning. He was told – this is what the crowds want. They want to see the fights.

That story has always stayed with me. I think about that as I watch two players dual and wonder how long it will be before the linesman steps in. It also makes me wonder about us – the fans. Is that what we really want? Is seeing fights on the ice better than watching excellent passing and scoring?

When I was young, hockey players did not wear helmets. I can remember the toothy grins most players had. And I remember the great Gordie Howe. Howe's wife, Colleen, died of Pick's Disease at the age of 79. After that, Howe was approached by Baycrest Hospital, to put his face on a fund-raising campaign for Alzheimer's. This is the same hospital I recently had some testing done at.

The eighth annual Scotiabank Pro-Am for Alzheimer's hockey tournament in support of Baycrest is scheduled for 2014. Hockey legends

Wendel Clark, Marcel Dionne and Doug Gilmour will be lacing up their skates in support. This tournament secures critical funds for Baycrest in support of Alzheimer's research. Baycrest's Rotman Research Institute is one of the top five brain institutes in the world, leading ground-breaking research to understand the mechanisms of memory and executive functions of the brain, in normal aging and in the presence of dementia, Alzheimer's, stroke and other conditions and diseases.

I know what its like to have a concussion. About 10 years ago, I hit the side of my head on our van door. I was not able to work for one month; I was nauseous; had migraine headaches; couldn't drive; couldn't look at things; saw white dots, etc. I was told by my doctor there was nothing I could do except wait it out. Sometimes I wonder if this is the reason, I now am cognitively impaired with dementia. Perhaps this will be determined at the time when my brain is donated to science.

It also makes me wonder how many athletes are put back into the game with a concussion. Of course, "they're tough... they can take it."

I'm now back to where I started: another hockey player received a concussion. Is this truly part of the good ole' hockey game? Or should we be ashamed of ourselves for encouraging the bashing of brains to the force of ultimately dementia?

The Fog

Date: October 6th, 2013

I have heard about The Fog many times. I have read about The Fog many times. But, I had yet to truly experience it. Today, that changed. I got lost in The Fog.

For those us with dementia, The Fog can help describe the feeling when your brain is not working to capacity. Words and memories can come and go depending on the thickness of The Fog.

I have had a terribly busy week and have pushed my brain hard to operate on all cylinders. Somewhat like a car battery, today I could feel my brain struggling as if it did not have a full charge. It was frustrating. Interesting enough, the weather today has been rainy and very foggy.

It seemed like the weather reflected my brain. It was hard to see, and lights did not give out a brightness but rather they were dim.

I took a walk tonight. I tried to understand what was going on. The road was dark with only some occasionally lite trailers. I thought of the analogy of my brain and this evening walk in the fog. Today, I struggled with finding words and naming things. I kept looking for them, but the words evaded me. It was just darkness. I looked for the moon to help light up the night so I could see more clearly where I was walking. The moon wasn't there. It was only The Fog.

I thought to myself, is this what it will be like when The Fog encloses in on me. Will the dim lights be my only source to charge my brain? Will this darkness lift allowing words to come into my brain?

In a good scary movie, many times fog rolls in creating an eerie atmosphere. It hides things and makes it hard to see what is coming. Today, it wasn't the fog of a movie that scared me – it was The Fog.

I now have joined the The Dementia Fog club. I must keep striving for the light.

Learning From my Peers

Date: October 19, 2013

A few weeks ago, I had an incredible experience. I meet three extraordinary peers while taping a new web video series titled "Through our eyes – *Living* with dementia." MAREP has asked director Chris Wynn to film the journey of the host (me) who is newly diagnosed with dementia. The film is made up of several different episodes where I meet others with dementia who have journeyed. Through the episodes, they share with me how to live well. Isn't that cool?!

Chris is renowned for his film Forgetful Not Forgotten, "...an intimate portrait of a family coming to grips with the realities of early-onset Alzheimer's disease."

The first episode takes place at our kitchen table. Dawn, Brianna, and I discuss our journey with dementia. Initially, I was very aware of the camera's and lights. I did my best to stay focused on my conversations. The interesting thing I have noticed is I don't really become nervous anymore. I'm excited but not nervous.

Filming a documentary means you don't have to remember lines. There are suggested topics to help guide the conversation. But other than that, the camera tries to capture the essence through non-rehearsed conversations. For someone like me, that's perfect. I did not feel pressure to say certain things. For those who may be a bit nervous, it allows freedom to converse freely as well.

My first meeting was with Brenda Hounam. Brenda and I already know each other from other projects. I consider Brenda to be my mentor. She has been key to initiate and complete several different potentially life changing projects. She is a pioneer in dementia advocacy. As always, it was wonderful to listen to her share key strategies to live well with dementia.

A few days later, the camera crew, Dawn and I met at Ron and Anne Hopewell's home. This was my first-time meeting Ron and Anne. Ron shared with me a wonderful book of photo's showing him building his home a few years ago in Quebec. Ron is immensely proud of his accomplishments – as he should be. As we stood on their balcony, he shared with me some his main points to live well with dementia. I listened carefully.

The final meeting was at Ron and Nora Hustwitt's home. Ron was standing at the door to welcome us in. His smile is contagious. The four of us talked while sitting at their kitchen table. Ron shared with me some of his tools to help him schedule his day and discussed various groups he belongs to. The end our meeting was highlighted by their daughters' family arriving. The three little ones chattered excitedly about being on film. What a wonderful, positive environment for anyone to live in!

The segment that I found to be the most exciting was the next one. All four of us met at the Village of Winston Park. It was then that I shared with me peers all the many things I had learned from them on my journey. It was interesting to see that as I spoke, for some, I was teaching them something new. I had come into the journey, thinking that my peers would tell me the same thing. But, just in a different fashion. This was not the case. Once again, never assume!

Our conversation then switched to what we can do to further our advocacy. It was amazing to be part of my peers and brainstorming ideas. I look forward to working with them on furthering these ideas to come to fruition.

The filming is not yet complete. Chris will be back to capture some more next month. Although this has been exciting to be a partner of, I have also found it tiring. I find the need to be "on." This pressure comes from myself not others.

MAREP has begun to advertise the video series premiere of "Through our eyes – *Living* with Dementia."

Once again, I find myself on another adventure. How can I not be *living* well with dementia?

Bill 356 & Bill 54

Date: October 26th, 2013

I thought I had a fairly good understanding on the political arena regarding national and provincial dementia strategies. Much to my embarrassment, I have discovered I know truly little about such important information.

Recently, I was discussing with some peers about possible ways we can advocate for an Ontario dementia plan. We came up with some wonderful ideas and next steps. While researching as part of the next steps, I discovered that Ontario already had a provincial plan. The 1999-2004 Alzheimer Strategy was the first of its kind in Canada.

How can I have not known about this? I find this to be disconcerting.

I continued my goggling and dug deeper into the internet abyss. Once again – to my surprise – Members Bill 54 (provincial) came into my line of Google results. Bill 54, Alzheimer Advisory Council Act, 2013 is a private members Bill. With the support of Progressive Conservative deputy leader Christine Elliott, Liberal MPP Donna Cansfield introduced the Bill for the third time in April 2013 and it received second reading in May 2013. It is an Act to establish the

Alzheimer Advisory Council and develop a strategy for the research, treatment and prevention of Alzheimer's disease and other forms of dementia. In its composition shall include persons with Alzheimer's disease or other forms of dementia.

I am so excited to find that there is something already in motion in Parliament. Also, it is great to see that the population that this Bill is about, is to be included in the makeup of the committee.

In a quick comparison between Bill 54 and the 1999-2004 Alzheimer's Strategy plan, it is heartening to see that we have come along way. The first plan did not include those with dementia within its committee makeup.

Continuing my quest for information regarding parliamentary dementia Bills, again I am surprised to learn that there is a Private Members Bill already introduced in the House of Commons. In 2011, MP Claude Gravelle put forth legislation for a national dementia strategy. In summary this enactment requires the Minister of Health to initiate discussions with the provincial and territorial ministers responsible for health or health promotion for the purpose of developing a national strategy for the health care of persons afflicted with Alzheimer's disease or other dementia-related diseases.

In addition to all of this, in July 2013 a meeting of the Council of the Federation's Health Care Innovation Working Group made dementia an important priority issue. The Premiers directed the Group to examine issues related to dementia, including identifying best practices for early diagnosis. Central to this is raising awareness of the early warning signs and various methods of intervention.

Although a bit red-faced in not knowing all the great things happening within Parliament, I am extremely happy in my new knowledge. I figure if I don't know this, there are more like me.

I wonder to myself how can this information be better disseminated so it reaches us regular folks. Because it is us regular folks who want to support these Bills. We will put our names on the petitions and demand from our government a national and provincial dementia strategy.

Get your pen out, a petition is coming soon to a place near you.

Attitude of Gratitude

November 15th, 2013

Imagine a world-wide poll asking individuals if they are living well. The answer is either yes or no. What percentage of us would respond yes? I'm a bit worrisome of the potential answer to the question.

Over the last few days, I have been mulling over possible topics for todays journal. I've been looking for a topic of inspiration. It has been a tough week for our world. At home, CBC News continues its coverage on crack-smoking Toronto mayor Rob Ford. To our neighbours in the south – the Obama Health Care Plan is trying to recover from a disastrous implementation. The Philippines desperately try to bring relief to Typhoon Haiyan victims. Shall I go on?

My answer to our hypothetical international poll is "Yes." I am living well – regardless of my dementia. I'm sure that the World Health Organization has a definition for living well. But for simplicity, use your own definition. What is your answer? I hope it was Yes.

This provides a nice segue into what I really want to write about: "Attitude of Gratitude." Today, I received an email from "A Meeting of the Minds" which connects people diagnosed with dementia and others who are meeting the challenges of dementia through videoconferencing. It is a one-of-a-kind inspiring monthly meeting hosted by Richard Taylor, PhD and Laura Bowley. In this months Cafe Le Brain, hosted by A Meeting of the Minds, participants are invited to share three things for which they are grateful and develop an "attitude of gratitude." Ahhh – perfect, I have found my topic!

When I take a step back and try and define and limit the number of things, I am grateful for, it is challenging. I have so many. I am grateful for my partner Dawn and daughter Brianna. For just about 13 years now, these two wonderful ladies have loved me unconditionally. They are my key to living-well and provide for me a solid foundation which channels my desire to be an advocate for those less fortunate than myself. The twinkles in their brown eyes remind me to live, love, and laugh.

I am grateful for my parents, family, and friends. My Mom and Dad demonstrate what a strong marriage is all about. While growing up, they encouraged me to love God, my family, and treat others as I wished to be treated. Being the last of 8 children, or the Baby, I am fortunate to have great individual relationships, with lots of nieces and nephews. I have in-laws who love me for who I am. I have been blessed with many friends over the years. I am so thankful for them and their influence on who I am today.

I am grateful for being Canadian and living in Canada. I have travelled around the world, and yes, there are many beautiful places, but I would never give up Canada for any of them. I have been able to live in peace without restrictions based on race, gender, religious beliefs, sexual orientation, and living with dementia.

I leave with some food for thought for you. Although these are troubled times, maybe it will be an interesting exercise for you to ask yourself to identify three things that you are grateful for. Once you get going, its hard to stop! And from this, we all can develop an "attitude of gratitude."

She Needs Wide Open Spaces

Date: November 27th, 2013

Our home seems quiet tonight. Dawn is busy at work; I'm puttering around, and Shiloh is asleep in his bed. The house also seems different – which it is.

This morning, Brianna, and her good friend Anna headed off to Port Elgin. They had two cats and a car stuffed full of items two young women need when they first move away from home. Yes, we are now experiencing the empty nest syndrome.

I remember my Mom telling me the older you get; the years go by that much faster. How true she was. It seems like yesterday when our little girl wanted a bedtime story to be read to her; she NEEDED a pony; wore braces; had her first job; cried when a boy hurt her heart; and sang with me songs from The Sound of Music.

Today, she was laughing, smiling and was excited about the new adventure. She was moving out. Dawn did her best to keep packing more and more things for the girls until there truly wasn't any more room. I focused on making sure she knew how to charge her car battery; had window fluid and could see out the back window of the car.

As we stood together on the porch waving goodbye, we commented on how excited we were for Brianna. It is time to spread her wings and fly. We can only hope that we have taught her "the right things" and have given her the self-confidence needed to stand on her own two feet. We hope that Brianna will work hard and strive to achieve the goals she sets for herself. We hope that she will be blessed by making good solid relationships which will help her in reaching her full potential. We hope for her happiness and love.

We will miss our baby girl. But we also look forward to watching her grow and accomplish all that she sets out to.

Tonight, I have been humming the Dixie Chicks song "Wide Open Spaces." It seems a fitting song for my mood.

We love you Bri. Enjoy your wide-open spaces! Xoxo

Neuropsychological Test

Date: December 4th 2013

I have never been one to excel in testing. Even from a young age, it seems like things freeze up on me. So, you can imagine how I must have felt this past Monday taking a test that lasted 6.5 hours.

Dawn, and our friend Shelley headed to Toronto on Sunday night so I could be well rested for our Monday 9:30 appointment at Baycrest Hospital. We met with Dr. Stokes and her test administrator for about an hour prior to testing. Dawn and the Doctor left the small testing room and I was left alone with the administrator. We were ready to begin.

Over the next 6.5 hours I would take neuropsychological tests which would assess and measure my cognitive function. Cognitive tests are vital in the diagnosis of dementia and may be used to differentiate between types of dementia.

The battery of test focus on major areas of cognition including:

- ✓ attention/concentration
- ✓ reasoning/conceptual shift
- ✓ verbal fluency
- ✓ language
- ✓ spatial processing
- ✓ immediate memory recall
- ✓ delayed memory recall
- ✓ delayed memory recognition
- ✓ expression of emotion

Neuropsychological tests are standardized. My individual scores would then be interpreted by comparing it to that of healthy individuals of a similar demographic background (i.e. Age, education, gender, etc.) and to expected levels of functioning. In this way, my doctor can determine whether my performance on any given task represents a strength or weakness. This in turn, would tell how my brain is functioning.

To give you some examples, tests for my language and speech skills included naming pictures my administrator showed me and name as many words as I could think of that began with a certain letter. To test my reasoning, planning, and organizing skills I was asked to sort cards according to colours or shapes on the cards. And I used a pencil to connect a series of numbered dots on a sheet of paper.

To test my attention span and memory I was asked to repeat a series of numbers and letters and words. I was also asked to look at a drawing and then draw it from memory.

I then began the "Wisconsin card sorting test." Initially, several cards were presented to me. I was then told to match the cards, but not how to match. I was only told if a match was right or wrong.

As I began the test, I thought there was something familiar about it. Finally, it occurred to me that this was the same test I take at lumosity. com. It forces me to think on my feet as rules change. Initially, I was very challenged and did not understand the test at Luminosity. I was frustrated by it, but persevered and became much better. I looked up at the Administrator and started to giggle which then turned into a full-out laugh. I triumphantly informed her I knew this test and could do it. If it were not for Luminosity, I know I would have easily failed this test. But, because I was familiar with it, I was able to quickly adapt to the rule changes. I'm sure I did very well.

After 6.5 hours, I had my shoes off and my head down on the table. I was told the testing was finished. Dr. Stokes and Dawn came back into the room. The Doctor thanked me for working so hard. My brain was mush and I was ready to go home.

I do not know how I did overall on the tests. There is no pass or fail – just a comparison to others. In the new year, the results will be shared with us.

If there is one thing I have learned, it is the importance of continuing to challenge myself with programs like Luminosity. It worked – which means I need to keep on working.

8115 Vilakazi Street, Soweto

Date: December 6th, 2013

It was August 1999, and I was working in one of the most dangerous cities of the world – Johannesburg, South Africa. I was there for three weeks, with a co-worker, training staff on new software.

From other co-workers I had been told terrifying stories of car jacking and hiding underneath blankets in the taxi so as not to be seen by passersby. Because of the danger, a young man everywhere escorted us. It is from this young black man; I was able to learn about the great Nelson Mandela.

Only two months earlier, South African President Nelson Mandela retired after serving his promised one term from 1994 – 1999. Mandela had served 27 years as a political prisoner before his release in 1990. Four years later he was inaugurated as South Africa's first black president in its first all-race election.

Looking out the car window, I watched the colourful people as we sped through the streets of Johannesburg and headed out of the city to the township of Soweto. The area was a mining belt. It also was formally an area where the government forced blacks to move outside legally designated white areas. This was done to help enforce the 1948 implementation of apartheid.

The effects of apartheid were still apparent. I only saw black faces. Whites did not live in Soweto.

Our young driver shared the stories of black resistance against minority rule which took place in this famous township. I could imagine the sights and sounds of violence as we drove through the streets to 8115 Vilakazi. We were heading to the house Mandela lived in before he went underground in the early 1960s. In 1997, this single-story red-brick house became a museum.

Walking up to the house, the feeling of history mixed with brutality and triumphs overcame me. We did not speak. Even after all these years, I could still feel the presence of this world hero, Nelson Mandela. The house remembered the dark days displaying bullet holes in the walls and scorch marks from attacks with Molotov cocktails.

It is humble home of three rooms with concrete floors. Original furnishings and memorabilia including photographs and citations cover the walls. I did my best to absorb the story the rooms were trying to tell me.

It is the story of a black man who was willing to die for his country fighting for the end of apartheid. It is the story of violence, death, brutality, and ignorance. But it is also the story of victory, perseverance, and strength. It left an indelible mark on me.

Mandela returned to this house after his release from prison in 1990. At a rally welcoming him home to Soweto his opening words were, "I have come home at last."

If these walls could talk – they would sing songs of happiness about its former tenant. And they would morn for the passing of a great man named Nelson Mandela.

YEAR THREE

Backbone of the Healthcare System?

Date: January 21st, 2014

I've been preoccupied today and have a heavy heart. Yesterday, I received an email from Robert (fictitious name) asking for my help. Him and his wife were moving into an apartment in their daughter's home. They are an older couple and his wife has dementia. Prior to them moving in, some renovations need to be done to accommodate their needs and for them to be comfortable.

Robert's question to me was if I knew if funding was available for the renovations. At this point, his daughter would have to personally finance the modifications. I sent him information on the program "Ontario Renovates" which is being delivered by the Region of Waterloo on behalf of the Federal and Provincial governments. The program has limited funding to assist qualified low to moderate-income households by providing funds to do home repairs and home modifications for persons with disabilities. To qualify for this program, the applicants must own the existing home and meet specific income and home value criteria.

Some facts about this Program:

- Maximum of $25,000 for repairs and accessibility modifications
- A promissory note is needed to secure funding up to $15,000
- Funding exceeding $15,000 requires a mortgage registered on title

- Loan does not need to be repaid if homeowner lives in home for 10 years
- Home must be valued at less than $318,508
- Total gross income of all households' members must be below specified amounts based on family size.

One more fact is the application form is 13 pages. These pages ask for incredible amount of information related to family finances. It details how much you are worth, right down to the last penny. Oh, and there is one short page for medical information.

My friend Robert told me that his daughter has been informed their income is too high and the home is valued above the cut-off amount. He stated: "if it was our income, they were interested in I think we would have a good chance of receiving some aid."

The sad truth is there is little in the way of finances available to help those with dementia and their family to help fund renovating their home. These renovations are necessary to be safe and comfortable in their own home. Robert is certainly not the first, nor will be the last, to be frustrated by a lack of consistent, readily- available information regarding this topic. I like him, am puzzled on why this grant looks at the family finances and not his own.

The Ontario Alzheimer has picked up on this challenge. It has asked the government to: "Provide flexible housing options and technology to help people living with dementia and other persons with accessibility challenges remain more independent."

On November 18th, 2013 I met with a group of my peers and caregivers. In that meeting we developed several points important to us and that we would like to see addressed within a provincial and national dementia plan. It included: "Financial assistance – to persons living with dementia and family partners in care."

For this to happen, the entire healthcare system must stop relying on family and friends to be the backbone of Canada's healthcare system. A mentality shift needs to occur before this vulnerable backbone becomes too stressed and financially drained to continue.

Australia and Denmark have proven through their National Home Care Strategy that it is possible. Other international models exist which do not rely on the family to be the primary health providers.

My friend Robert is like so many others. He does not know what services are available. What is unnerving is that an increase in Canadians over the age of 65 living at home with dementia is expected to rise from 55% to 62% by 2038. (Alzheimer Society of Canada, 2008).

I hopefully have a few more years before any home modifications need to be made for me. During this time, I can only look to the government and our healthcare leaders to work with us in developing and implementing a strategy that works.

In the meantime, my thoughts are with Robert and his family as they grapple with the struggles of living with dementia.

Sochi 2014

Date: February 7th, 2014

Today the world, with all its media, turns to the coastal city Sochi, Russia. The Olympic Winter Games opening ceremony is beginning to parade the 88 nations involved in this much anticipated event.

For me, the Olympics is a wonderful way to combine my strong national Canadian pride with my love of sports and its athletes. From a young age, I have been much interested in this international event. For my speech in grade five, I shared with my classmates the details of the Ancient Olympic games – the precursor for our modern Olympics featuring summer and winter games.

For my next year's speech, I once again turned to the Olympics and told the inspirational tale of American athlete, Wilma Rudolph. She was considered the fastest woman in the 1960s and competed in two Olympic games in 1956 and 1960. She won three gold medals in a single Game and earned the nickname "The Black Pearl." I wrote about her because I found her to be inspirational. Rudolph contracted infantile paralysis, recovered, but wore a brace on her leg until she was nine. For another two years she wore a special shoe. During that time, she also survived bouts of polio and scarlet fever. My young mind dreamed of how I could become a professional basketball player. Rudolph taught me that anything was possible.

My love for history combined with my love for the Olympics has taught me that unfortunately, it isn't all about sports. The 1936 Summer Olympics was held in Berlin, Germany. Initially, the Nazi party promoted that Jews and Black people should not be allowed to participate in the Games. Faced with a boycott of other nations, Hitler allowed for them to join the Games. Instead, the Nazi's banned non-Aryan from Germany's Olympic team, except for one German woman who had a Jewish father.

The Sochi Olympics has been shrouded in serious concerns of safety for its athletes, its audience and news of costs over-run, corruption, anti-gay propaganda laws, hotels un-ready, etc., etc. All forms of social media is being used to feed into this frenzy of bashing this event.

As I watch the opening ceremonies on television, I am grateful for speakers who are reminding all of us about what the Olympics is about - the best athletes in the world coming together to compete. Finally! Perhaps the world is now ready to switch its attention to our nations heroes as everyone strives to be all they can.

In 2012, my nephew Jason had the wonderful opportunity to attend the summer Olympics in London. He and his wife Theresa were in the stands to cheer on her sister – a Canadian Olympian – Sheila Reid. I felt excitement for the Reid family. It must be something to be privy to watching an Olympian grow up and ultimately compete in an event for which they trained for most of their lives. Jason took breath taking photo's capturing the essence of the Games. I stayed glued to the television to cheer on someone I knew. Sheila's' journey was inspiring.

The world needs heroes. For someone like me who has dementia, they remind me that I can accomplish goals I set out for myself – even if they seem unachievable. I always like the underdog who clamors to stand on the podium. It is somewhat like the dementia population as we strive to be on a podium to have our voices heard. We just keep working, a step at a time.

The Olympic Movement which through the Olympic rings reinforces the idea that it is international and welcomes all countries of the world to join. I will be one of millions of viewers excited to see the athletes live up to the Olympic motto "Citius, Altius, Fortius" which is Latin for "Faster, Higher, Stronger." I wish the best to each Olympian. They have worked hard and have given up much to be the best in the world. And for the 221 Canadian's – Go Team, Go!

The End of Banking

Date: February 12th, 2014

Mathematician is not a word that describes me. Even as far back as kindergarten, I struggled with simple arithmetic such as 1 + 1. It rarely seemed to add to 2. Thank goodness for the calculator for which I have relied upon to perform these mathematical feats.

At the time of my diagnosis of probable Frontotemporal Lobe dementia (FTD), we were told to get my affairs in order. Furthermore, it was suggested to Dawn that she keeps my credit and bank cards. The reasoning is that dementia leads to deficits in functional abilities. This translates into me being challenged by complex tasks such as bill paying, working, shopping, managing appointments, etc.

We've known for years I had been making poor decisions with the family finances, resulting in a huge hit to it. This is typical in patients with bvFTD. My poor judgement and impulsivity have placed my family at financial risk.

This intervention by care partners, is essential to prevent overspending. With that said, it did not make it easier to hand over my credit card and my bank card (even though I was always forgetting my pin number). For the past 1 1/2 years, we have been living this way. I can keep a few dollars in my wallet to spend. When my money runs out, I ask Dawn if I can have some more. I'm asked what the money is for prior to receiving it.

You can imagine the feeling I may experience going through this process. In my brain, I know this is the right thing to do, but it still stings my independence streak.

The one banking task I have continued with is paying the bills. How much trouble can I get into doing that? Well, let me tell you.

Two weeks ago, we received a notice in the mail, that we had not paid our hydro bill. We would be cut off if it weren't done immediately. It was a shock to receive such a bill. How can I have missed doing that? Somehow, I did.

Just this week, I used on-line banking to pay our bills. This is a normal job for me. We have an account which we dedicate to for such expenses which holds just enough money to cover the bills. At the end of the session, I reviewed what I had done, and realized I made a few mistakes. The first is, I over-paid a bill by $250. The second mistake, I did not pay one of the bills and now did not have enough money in the account to do so. And the third mistake, I brought our account into the negatives by making the previous mistake.

As I pondered my actions, sadness overtook me. I know I am no longer capable to properly pay the bills. I called Dawn over to my side and showed her my banking mistakes. I told her "I can't pay the bills anymore." Without missing a beat, she suggested that we do this task together. In that flash of a moment, she made me feel better about not being able to do the banking. We will do it as a team. Just like we have done all things during our 12 years of being together.

When I made the decision to share my journey through writing journals, I knew that I did not want to shy away from difficult topics. To do so, only leads to further stigma and shrouds dementia.

I can still live well – even without executing the family bill paying. Dawn has once again reinforced her love and support for me, by having us do this task as a couple.

Many times, I receive the comment, "Gee, you don't look/act like you have dementia." Rest assured, I have it. It just took another kick at my independence.

Technology

Date: February 21st, 2014

This past week, I somehow managed to wreck our microwave, rendering it useless. For me, I did not have an immediate need to go out and purchase one. The "old fashion" way of heating things up on the stove, was simply fine. What struck me as funny, was Brianna's reaction to the loss of this appliance: "How do you warm up food?" "On the stove??!" "We need to get a new microwave!" Yesterday, Brianna did just that – she went out to the store and bought our new microwave.

Brianna's reaction to not having a microwave makes me chuckle. It also reminds me of when my Mom bought her first microwave. As she put it proudly on the kitchen counter, we asked her "What do you do with it?" "You mean we don't warm our food up on the stove?"

Technology is an interesting thing. It seems as fast as something is developed, there is a newer, better, faster, more efficient model right behind. When I was grade 4, my Mom was a legal secretary. For her job, she sometimes brought homework to finish up. To do this, she also brought home an electric typewriter. Well... didn't I think we were the coolest! I remember the loud hum of the machine as it was turned on. My Mom would put me in front of it with a piece of paper and instructed the sentence I was to type. How I loved the sound of the clicking as I tapped the keys.

Fast-forward to today. I have been doing my best to keep up with technology and use it to my advantage. About half a year ago, I created a Twitter account. Frankly, I still don't really understand this whole tweet thing. I muddle my way through re-tweets (RT) and hash tags. I am always amazed when I get a new follower. How do they find me? And of course, how do I get more followers?!

In addition to tweeting, over the last few months I have spent a great deal of time on YouTube. I love it and can spend hours on it in anyone sitting. I am always a sucker for funny animal videos. These videos can make me laugh hard – which is always good for the soul.

This past week, I participated in "A Meeting of the Minds" an online conference of people with dementia. The goal is to "...inspire and enable people with dementia to help themselves and each other, and to bring people together in community." Using my computer, I was able to view and speak with people living with dementia from Montreal, Texas, Hawaii, England, and other far off cities. Together, it created a sense of community and camaraderie.

I have been pondering on how to use technology, YouTube, to help in my advocacy work of living well with dementia. Originally, I was part of a team considering the creation and management of an international e-newsletter. We have started the project and have determined we wish to change the media format from an e-newsletter to short YouTube videos.

I envision it looking something like this: Each week I will video tape myself asking a question to our target audience of those living with dementia. The weekly question will be internationally appropriate and attempt to draw out comments, reactions, emotions, laughter, and camaraderie. In response to the weekly question, we will invite those living with dementia to respond using a short video limited to two minutes in length.

There is much power to be able to see a peer speaking. Perhaps the person may struggle a bit with word finding or lose their train-of-thought. It really doesn't matter. They are participating and thus, living well with dementia. For those who just wish to view the videos, it is a wonderful manner to listen to viewpoints from around the world on a subject. This helps in creating understanding, knowledge, and generate ties to a community. For those living in rural areas of the world, this is particularly useful.

One of the best YouTube videos I have seen comes from Waverly Mansion Retirement Residence located in London, Ontario. The Recreation Coordinator, Sarah Urquhart, works with the residents to produce uplifting videos using music. The elderly residents on video are singing, dancing, smiling, and laughing. Its infectious.

I think we all have something to learn from the Waverly residents and Ms. Urquhart. Technology can inspire and uplift our spirits. We just must do it.

The Suitcase

Date: February 27th, 2014

It was March 28th, 1923 at the Prince's Dock, Glasgow, Scotland. My Grandma Wighton, then known as Miss Bessie Thomson, was a 20-year-old single woman waiting to board the Cassandra. She had a ticket for Third class passage on this ship which would take her to the new world – Canada. It would take them a total of 21 days to cross the ocean and arrive at Pier 56, New York, USA. Once she arrived, a letter from her sister Lottie would be delivered to her. It would tell her "... take a taxi from the boat to the station in New York and make sure you won't lose yourself." She would follow her big sisters' directions which brought her safely to Toronto.

My family is fortunate to have an incredible article which she carried on this voyage. It is a wooden suitcase with a warn leather handle, dove tail corners, and finishing nails. There is no indication of what may have been housed in it. When opened, it smells of old wood and is barren. Its age – at least 91 years old.

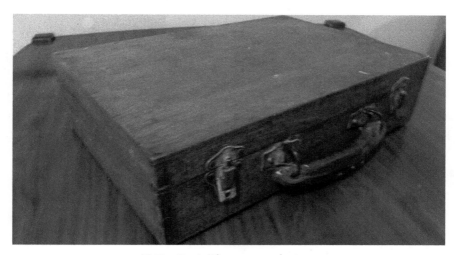

1923 - Bessie Thomson wood suitcase

My mind wanders off trying to imagine this incredible journey. I keep looking at the suitcase for clues of what it may have held. There are none. How difficult it must have been to decide what to put in this wooden box. Was its photo's? Letters? Special clothing? We will never know.

Lately, I have been working on a few projects which focuses on "after diagnosis" of my dementia. Just like my Grandma, I too am on a journey of leaving my old world and life and am now part of a new world, with dementia. It is uncharted territory and there are many new people coming into my life and new things to be learned.

I ask myself: If I was able to use the same wooden suitcase which my Grandma used for her journey, what would I put in it? What possessions from my past do I value the most? What articles can help me in this journey of dementia? My bible? Is it pictures? Old letters? Awards of recognition? Small mementos?

That's the funny thing about both our journey's – it is all guess work on what can help us and comfort us. I would imagine my Grandma would have looked to others to help her if she did not find what she needed in her wooden suitcase. It has seen 91 years of history and holds many stories.

Perhaps someday far off in the future, someone will open my suitcase and my journey will unfold. What it will say, I do not know. We will just have to wait and see.

iPod Music Therapy

Date: March 4th, 2014

It is probably about the year 1971. I am five years old and am at my best friend Lori's house. Lori had received a set of drums for Christmas and I was giving them a heck of a workout. Lori was singing her heart out to our audience – her Mom and a sister.

I joined her in the lines I knew: "Jeremiah was a bull frog. Was a good friend of mine. Never understood a single word he said but I helped him drink his wine." And then I would proceed with some drumming. You may recognize this song as "Joy to the World" from Three Dog Night made in 1971.

Fast forward three years. Lori and I are running in the park across from my house. At the top of our lungs we are singing "In the heat of the summer night; in the land of the dollar bill; when the town of Chicago died; and they talk about it still...nahhnaah..." My transistor radio blared this popular 1971 Paper Lace song "The Night Chicago Died."

It's a strange thing – I can remember many songs from when I was quite young yet can't remember anything about a movie, I watched last week. I am not the only one. As you are probably well-aware, music can bring us back to times of long ago.

A new documentary titled "Alive Inside: A Story of Music and Memory" follows a social worker named Dan Cohen who has launched a campaign to bring iPods and music therapy to nursing homes. One of the central characters he works with is a 90-year-old Alzheimer's patient named Henry. He was featured in a video posted online that went viral in 2012 with over 10 million viewers.

The video begins with Henry looking largely unresponsive. Then he was given a pair of headphones to listen to Cab Calloway, his favorite artist. Suddenly, he is singing and moving to the music.

There is a great deal of research and evaluation of music with dementia patients. It shows consistent results: residents are happier, more social, and calmer. Largely due to these findings, "iPod projects" are now available at many different locations and through several associations. Close to home, the Alzheimer society of London and Middlesex have posted on their website information on how to soon participate in this program.

On a personal level, I am interested in this program. A dear friend of mine, who is nearly mute with Alzheimer's, will soon be starting the iPod music therapy program. I believe one of the first steps is to discover her favorite music. I hope this therapy will get her toes tapping and bring her back to a place in her memories of happiness.

For me, I have been wondering what music I will put on my iPod. For sure, it will include "Jeremiah was a bull frog" and "The Night Chicago Died."

The Window to the Soul

Date: March 7th, 2014

I have not had the pleasure to be in the same room as the Mona Lisa picture. But I have enjoyed looking at this interesting picture through books and replicas. I am like millions of others who have experienced the feeling that her eyes seem to follow you wherever you go. It is a curious feeling. Supposedly, it has something to do with the way it is painted and a lack of third dimension of the canvas.

Eyes. There are so many ways to describe eyes: She has a twinkle in her eye; His eyes are dark and mysterious; His eyes look sad; She has a gleam in her eyes and his eyes are soulless.

Audrey Hepburn was quoted: "The beauty of a woman must be seen from in her eyes, because that is the doorway to her heart, the place where love resides." And how many times have you heard the proverb to "never trust anyone who can't look you in the eyes?" And the famous saying: "The Eyes are the window to your soul."

I always have been sensitive to the look into people's eyes. I really do believe they are the "window to your soul." I think they tell us things that our mouth doesn't or is incapable.

I believe my own eyes have taken on a look of sadness. A very dear friend of mine has recently progressed into the end stages of Alzheimer's. Recently, I went to visit her, and I looked deeply into her eyes. Her eyes are a beautiful colour of blue and grey and they will twinkle when she is happy. Sadly, the twinkle is gone, and it's been replaced by the look of fogginess.

She no longer says my name as she is nearly mute. And when I look into her eyes, I don't believe they recognize me for a cloudiness takes over. Regardless, I hold her hand and tell her how much I love her.

I wonder where she goes when that blank look takes over. She obviously is not here. I wonder if this is when her soul has started to go towards heaven. Perhaps she is in a middle place where she comes and goes. It brings me comfort to know that when her soul does go to heaven, she will have her twinkle back for the rest of eternity.

The Waverley Mansion Grandchildren

March 21st, 2014

I needed a bit of an "ump" today. Although the sun is shining and I saw a Robin, I was still in need of something to get me smiling.

I found it through YouTube. Sarah Urquhart, the Recreation Coordinator of Waverley Mansion located in London, Ontario, filmed and directed the teaming up of Waverley Mansion Retirement Residents and their Waverley Grandchildren. This inter-generational group sang, danced, and acted to Hedley's song "I Can Do Anything."

I just love it! Love it! Love it! When watching the YouTube video, you can't help but smile and start to hum along with the song. Previous songs created by Ms. Urquhart and the Residents have them dancing and singing. Through this process, stigma is broken down and positive education occurs.

With this latest video, the addition of the Residents Grandchildren makes the video all that more endearing and once again breaks down the walls of stigma.

It is a clear message these wonderful videos send us. Just because you live in a retirement home and have grey hair, doesn't mean you can't sing, dance, laugh and have fun. By including their grandchildren in the video with them, once again it breaks down stigma that older people are boring and are always sick, fragile, and lay in bed all day.

I remember visiting my Grandma at an old age home. Many of the residents would sit in the front room. They looked forlorn. I didn't like the smell of the home as it seemed stale. I don't remember any inter-generational projects which would have helped with reducing stigma and provided opportunities for me to have fun with my Grandma.

As Canadian retirement homes continue to look for ways to improve, I do hope they are taking lessons from the Residents of Waverley and Ms. Urquhart. It is for sure that their Grandchildren will have a much different perspective of a retirement home than I did at their age. Well-done!

A Changing Melody 'Life Beyond Diagnosis"

Date: May 15th, 2014

A few weeks ago, I had the honour and pleasure to be the Keynote speaker at A Changing Melody forum in St. Catherines, Ontario. This was a day of learning and sharing for Persons with early-stage dementia and their Partners in Care.

For 50 minutes I discussed and shared information about three main topics:

✓ The Dementia Movement
✓ A call to advocacy, and
✓ Advocacy projects I'm involved in.

I was quite moved by the standing ovation I received from my peers, friends, and others.

While answering questions from the audience, I was amazed at the many individuals who was not aware of some of the points I was sharing. Many did not know Canada and Ontario does not have a dementia plan. This was a strong reminder of the importance of education and not assuming others have all the information everybody needs.

The room was full of raw energy. People wanted to know where someone may sign petitions and how to act as advocates for those with dementia. It was obvious the participants did not want to sit back and let others do the work but instead, they wanted to help. It was a wonderful sight!

I love the story of how A Changing Melody was named. During a 1995 performance by violinist Itzhak Perlman, one of the strings on his violin broke. The audience could hear the loud snap. Without hesitating he continued to play, changing, and recomposing the pieces as he went. When he finished, people rose and cheered to show their appreciation for what he had done. It was then Perlman said to the audience: "You know, sometimes it is the artist's task to find out how much music he can still make with what he has left."

If you are someone with a diagnosis of dementia, it is easy to relate to the symbolism of this story. The breaking of the string on the violin is the time of diagnosis. It is at this time, we are forced to decide on how we wish to live our lives – or, continue to play the violin.

We may change the melody we play by focusing on the abilities and talents we still possess, instead of playing Overture to William Tell, perhaps we will switch to Handels Hallelujah Chorus or Beethoven's 5th Symphony. We can still play intense, passionate, beautiful music.

When our symbolic violin string breaks, we then transition to "life beyond diagnosis." You then must decide on how to live. For me, I could accept and embrace the diagnosis, or I could choose to reject it and live in anger and with sadness. It was an easy decision to embrace it. I changed when I was diagnosed. I decided to be an advocate for those with dementia.

On the drive home from the forum, Dawn and our friend Shelley chatted about the day. I reflected on how blessed I am. I have people in my life who want to help me live well after my diagnosis. Once again, we embraced carpe diem and had a wonderful adventure.

The Dementia Movement

Date: May 21st, 2014

I love history. I enjoy hearing the stories of where we came from and the struggles the pioneers overcame so that we may live a wonderful life.

Today, I will be discussing some of the key historical moments of the Dementia Movement.

When I think of the word "Movement" I think of a powerful social challenge to the current status quo. Wikipedia defines a social movement as: "A coordinated group action focused on a political or social issue." Think of it as the uprising and protest that changes the course of history.

Wikipedia cites a long list of movements including:

✓ Anti-apartheid movement
✓ Anti-bullying movement
✓ Civil rights
✓ Children's rights
✓ Human rights
✓ Women suffrage movement, and the recent
✓ Occupy Wall Street.

There are many more on this list. But what isn't on this list is the "Dementia Movement." At least not yet!

You may be thinking, I've never heard of the "Dementia Movement." Rest assured, there is a movement, and it is slowly rumbling from a whisper to louder and louder.

For those of us diagnosed with dementia, the year 2000 is of great significance for it is when Lorraine Smith created on Yahoo "The Dementia Advocacy and Support Network" (DASNI) for early-stage dementia and their care partners.

It was in the year 2001, when 12 of the 82 members of DASNI, came together in Montana and DASNI International was formed. Further to that, Christine Bryden was the first person in the world with a diagnosis to present at a major international conference. This was the first-time people with dementia attended the international conference as full participants.

With Bryden's brilliant speech and the active attendance by the other 12 participants with dementia, it sent a message to the international community that people with dementia showed irrefutably that not only does life continue after diagnosis, but also that people with dementia have much to offer. The Dementia Movement began!

Creation of a Movement

When discussing the creation of a movement, you need to ask the question: "What needs to be changed?"

For those of us with dementia, there are several things such as:

✗   Canada does not have a National Dementia Plan to make dementia a public health priority.

✗   Ontario does not have a Provincial Dementia Plan to make dementia a public health priority.

✗   There is a lack of local services enabling us to live if possible, in our homes.

✗   There is a lack of adequate funding to support our families and careers to help them look after us if they can.

✗   There is a lack of adequate funding in the healthcare system to ensure appropriate dementia care and support when we need it.

✗   Everyone caring for us does not have training in person-centered care.

✗ Anti-psychotic drugs are not always used appropriately.

✗ We are not always part of our own end-of-life strategy plans.

✗ There is stigma and a lack of education, and

✗ We are not given a clear diagnosis early in the disease.

I'm sure each one of you also has a few points of your own which can be added to this list.

We have come a long way since the formation of DASNI in the year 2000. Many people have worked persistently and with enthusiasm to push for the rights of those with dementia. Because of the work of these pioneers, it is much easier to live well with dementia. We have a lot to thank them for.

I believe the Dementia Movement is picking up steam as more of us are advocating for our own rights and the rights of others. If I can quote Bob Dylan's political cry, "the times they are a-changing."

The Dementia Movement needs to win over neutrality, opinions and support of the populace and involve them in the process of opposition and change. We are doing that one step at a time!

Gone Fish'en

Date: June 14, 2014

It was so eerie. I loved it!

The fog rolled up the Saugeen river to meet the fog rolling in from Lake Huron. It happened so quickly that the sail boats and large commercial fishing boats disappeared in a matter of minutes. I could still hear voices from across the river but no longer saw the faces to go with them. The foghorn started to blare its warning every few minutes.

We were at my favorite fishing hole.

It's been about a month since I started my new hobby – fishing. We live in a town in which everyone seems to have a fishing pole and strategies to catch "the big one." I listen attentively to them in the hope that I can reproduce them.

So far, the "big one" has eluded me. Well, even just a little one has steered clear of all my different lures. Yup – not ta – skunked.

For some, this would be enough to throw the fishing pole in the water never to be used again. But not so for me. I absolutely love just sitting in my chair and enjoy the sights and sounds.

Although I love this new past-time, I also have found it a bit frustrating. And it's not for the lack of catching a fish. I struggle to remember the name of the fish that I want to catch. Is it trout, bass, or walleye? Depending on the type of fish, there are certain lures to use. I can't remember which lure goes with which fish. If the river is clear or cloudy, this is another variable that affects what I put on my line. There are simply too many variables and names for my short-term memory to retain.

In the first week of fishing, I lost several prize lures. I struggled to tie a proper fisherman's knot in the heat of the moment. Much to my dismay, I would watch them travel like a baseball and then hear the loud "plop."

I have come to the realization, that I'm a fishing-person who has dementia. The many things to remember to do and how to do it, I can't retain in my memory for as long as I need it. I decided that I have two choices: 1) not fish or 2) change how I fish. Number two is the winner.

The first modification was to make sure that I always have two fishing rods all rigged up before leaving the house. I no longer monkey around on the docks with trying different lures and struggle with making a good knot. If one gets snagged, I simply can switch my rod. This is now going much smoother.

While I am at home getting my rod ready, I have started to wear my new reading glasses. This has made a huge difference in that I can see what I'm doing. I also have a picture of the knot in front of me while I'm making my knots and give myself plenty of time to do it. I'm happy to say I have not lost any more lures.

My tackle box presents many challenges to me. I forget when, why and how to use the assortment of hooks, worms, lures, weights, etc. Today, I have come up with a solution. I bought a Fishing magazine containing lots of pictures. I plan to line my box with pictures and labels. That should help quite a bit.

Fishing is meant to be a peaceful activity. I don't want it to be stressful because I'm cognitively challenged.

At the end of the day, I could just sit in my chair with one rod and one lure and enjoy my surroundings.

And the fish? They better watch out because I'm coming for them!

The Long & Winding Road

Date: June 19th, 2014

In November 2013, in partnership with Murray Alzheimer Research and Education (MAREP), a group of individuals living with dementia and their care partners, came together to discuss the lack of both an Ontario and national dementia strategy plans. Conversations were guided using the philosophy "Nothing about Us without Us." The primary goal of the meeting was to educate, create, and document recommendations which will significantly enhance the lives of those living with dementia and care partners.

Listed below is the first point of this list of 10 points developed by this group. It targets the diagnosis experience.

"Improve the diagnosis experience. This can be accomplished through/by:

- Testing experiences
- Shorten length of time between assessments / testing
- Timely follow-up after diagnosis from professionals
- Acknowledge remaining skills/ strengths / capabilities
- Driving license removal progress – needs to be re-evaluated
- Improved sensitivity during communication of diagnosis to persons living with dementia and family partner in care. "

What is important to note is this challenging diagnosis experience is not specific to Canada. Across the globe, people with dementia are challenged by a long and winding road to diagnosis. For those with Younger Onset, this is particularly a great obstacle.

To demonstrate the need for an improvement of the diagnosis experience, I will use myself as the example.

From the year 2009 – today, I have been diagnosed with approximately 12 different diagnosis'. They are:

- PTSD
- Major Depression
- Forgetfulness
- No short-term memory impairment
- Probable Frontemporal dementia
- Frontal lobe problems

- OCD
- Panic Attacks
- Conversion Disorder
- Over-reporting of memory complaints
- Pituitary cyst

- REM sleep Behaviour disorder

This July, one more diagnosis will be added to my list. For the last two years, I have had body twitching. Although, I always tell my doctors about this twitching, it is not until now that it is being followed up on. I have an appointment in Toronto at Sunnyside hospital. I will be tested for ALS or Lou Gehrig's disease. It is a motor neuron disease. If I am positive for it, things will become that much more difficult for me.

Getting back to our discussion point of improvement of the diagnosis experience, let's talk about shortening the length of time between testing and timely follow-up by doctors. From May 2011, until now I have been through several tests including:

- MRI's
- MMSE's
- SPECT
- EEG
- Beck Depression Inventory
- MOCA's
- Sleep Test
- Neuropsychological Testing

I can give various examples of doctors not following up with us to discuss results of testing. Fortunately, my partner in care, Dawn, is excellent at contacting them and finding out the results. There are other examples of doctors asking us the results for tests as their peers did not follow through. It can be months of waiting before we hear the results.

Driver license removal process. For me, along with my diagnosis of FTD, I was told simply, "You cannot drive effective immediately." This is because of poor decision making. It seems to me there might be other more sensitive ways to communicate this. On the opposite side, some people should have their license revoked, yet it isn't. It is then left up to the family to try and negotiate with the person with dementia to not drive for they are unsafe to others and themselves.

Finally, "Improved sensitivity during communication of diagnosis to persons living with dementia and family partner in care." I exercised my right and obtained copies from my GP of all documentation on file for me. This is where you find the "real comments" from the doctors. Most patients do not actually read what their reports say. I strongly suggest that you do. It is within your medical file, comments from doctors can either positively or negatively affect your health insurance.

Once again, I'll use me as the example. The following comments are taken directly from my medical file or said to me:

"I honestly believe this is all psychiatric."

"I think Mary has adopted a sick role to not deal with her humiliations and to punish herself."

"There is no genuine memory problem and the issue is entirely emotional."

"If you do have dementia, it is game over!"

"Get your affairs in order."

During these past years, the focus from the medical community has been on what I can't do – not what I can still do. It is only through my own resolve and my partner Dawn's that we have striven to live carpe diem and not live in doom and gloom.

I recently was asked if I wasn't tired of all the doctors, tests, and diagnoses. I am. If it weren't for the demands by my private health insurance to continue with this, I'm not sure I would.

So, the next time someone suggests to you that we must improve the dementia diagnosis experience, I hope you remember me – and the story I told of the long and winding road.

Backbone of the Healthcare System?

Date: January 21st, 2014

I've been preoccupied today and have a heavy heart. Yesterday, I received an email from Robert (fictitious name) asking for my help. Him and his wife were moving into an apartment in their daughter's home. They are an older couple, and his wife has dementia. Prior to them moving in, some renovations need to be done to accommodate their needs and for them to be comfortable.

Robert's question to me was if I knew if funding was available for the renovations. At this point, his daughter would have to personally finance the modifications. I sent him information on the program "Ontario Renovates" which is being delivered by the Region of Waterloo on behalf of the Federal and Provincial governments. "The program has limited funding to assist qualified low to moderate-income households by providing funds to do home repairs and home modifications for persons with disabilities. To qualify for this program, the applicants must own the existing home and meet specific income and home value criteria."

Some facts about this Program:

- Maximum of $25,000 for repairs and accessibility modifications
- A promissory note is needed to secure funding up to $15,000
- Funding exceeding $15,000 requires a mortgage registered on title
- Loan does not need to be repaid if homeowner lives in home for 10 years
- Home must be valued at less than $318,508
- Total gross income of all households' members must be below specified amounts based on family size.

One more fact is the application form is 13 pages. These pages ask for incredible amount of information related to family finances. It details how much you are worth, right down to the last penny. Oh, and there is one short page for medical information.

My friend Robert told me that his daughter has been informed their income is too high and the home is valued above the cut-off amount. He stated if "it was our income they were interested in I think we would have a good chance of receiving some aid."

The sad truth is there is little in the way of finances available to help those with dementia and their family to help fund renovating their home. These renovations are necessary in order to be safe and comfortable in their own home.

Robert is certainly not the first, nor will be the last, to be frustrated by a lack of consistent, readily- available information regarding this topic. I like him, am puzzled on why this grant looks at the family finances and not his own.

The Ontario Alzheimer has picked up on this challenge. It has asked the government to: "Provide flexible housing options and technology to help people living with dementia and other persons with accessibility challenges remain more independent."

On November 18th, 2013 I met with a group of my peers and caregivers. In that meeting we developed several points important to us and that we would like to see addressed within a provincial and national dementia plan. It included: "Financial assistance – to persons living with dementia and family partners in care."

For this to happen, the entire healthcare system must stop relying on family and friends to be the backbone of Canada's healthcare system. A mentality shift needs to occur before this vulnerable backbone becomes too stressed and financially drained to continue.

Australia and Denmark have proven through their National Home Care Strategy that it is possible. Other international models exist which do not rely on the family to be the primary health providers.

My friend Robert is like so many others. He does not know what services are available. What is unnerving is that an increase in

Canadians over the age of 65 living at home with dementia is expected to rise from 55% to 62% by 2038.

I hopefully have a few more years before any home modifications need to be made for me. During this time, I can only look to the government and our healthcare leaders to work with us in developing and implementing a strategy that works.

In the meantime, my thoughts are with Robert and his family as they grapple with the struggles of living with dementia.

Carpe Diem at its Best

Date: July 8th, 2014

If you had a terminal illness, would you still live where you are currently? *Why* do you live where you do? Perhaps it is because you are close to your family; love your house; proximity to your job; or simply because that's where you have always lived.

If you were terminal, do those same reasons carry the same weight for staying? From my own experience, I can tell you "no" they do not.

For many years, Dawn, Brianna and I have vacationed in the beautiful town of Southampton located on Lake Huron. This quaint town is known for the best sunsets in Canada, beaches, fishing, birdwatching, lighthouses, canoeing, etc. In fact, in 2010, Chantry Island just off the coast of Southampton, was the winner for "Canada's Best Hidden Travel Gems."

It seems that every trip from our holiday town back to the "city" seems more and more difficult. We just love the peace and tranquility this area brings to us. Don't get me wrong, we also really enjoy our home, the area we live in, and the friendships we have developed. But we have seriously questioned if we wish to live in Kitchener any longer.

It was about two months ago when Dawn and I made the big decision to move from our security to the town of our dreams. After creating a list of pro's and con's, it was obvious that we both felt we would be happier in Southampton. Dawn has a home office which gives her the ability to work anywhere. My specialists are in Toronto which means we need to drive there regardless of where we live. I will not be changing any doctors. We do not have family here but do have some close friends. We will miss those friends dearly, but we know we will also develop new ones.

The last two months have been a whirlwind. We have decided to rent our home beginning in two weeks! We believe our renter will be a good fit for the neighborhood and be respectful of our property.

A few days ago, we secured our own place to rent. It is a small bungalow with everything on one floor. Exactly what we want. More importantly, the location is perfect for me to be able to walk to a few stores and of course Tim Horton's. Where we currently live, we are too far for me to walk to stores.

Because my license was revoked, I have been dependent on others. This move will provide me with the most independence I've had in two years. Further to that, a 20-minute walk will bring us right to the lake across from Chantry Island. This is a magical island that is a bird sanctuary and has an imperial tower lighthouse.

I have already scoped out possible volunteer positions. I think I'd like to try my hand at the Bruce County Museum & Cultural Centre. It has many possible opportunities to consider. Along with permanent exhibitions, it currently has a dinosaur one with all those old bones! Furthermore, it is just down the street from our new residence.

Also, down the street is a beautiful old church which we look forward to becoming members. And just pass that is an outdoor band stand located at the edge of a small lake. That's for Sunday evening entertainment. During the summer Sunday's evenings, a lone piper pipes down the sunset on the beach. My Scottish roots are excited!

As far as our family goes, they will still have to drive to come and see us. And that's OK. Brianna is currently living in Port Elgin just a stone throws away. She's not sure she'll stay there, but we can always hope!

Dawn and I have decided to be pro-active in putting in place a plan that allows us both to live well. If need be, an excellent hospital is right there as well as a long-term care facility.

We have heard and know of many people who are extremely financially strained due to the costs associated with dementia. People lose their homes. By this move, we put ourselves in a sound financial place. That means one less thing to worry about.

Reader, I ask you one more time – *why* do you live where you do? Perhaps you would like to join us in living carpe diem at its best.

Freedom!

Date: Aug. 1st 2014

Sometimes we do not realize all that we have until it is suddenly taken from you.

When I was diagnosed with probable Frontemporal Dementia (FTD) in September 2012, my driver's license was revoked effective immediately. The doctor informed me that having FTD made for poor decision making. Not only did I have to try and comprehend my terminal diagnosis, but I also had to come to terms with the loss of independence which my license provided to me.

Over the past two years, I have tried very hard not to complain about this loss. I try not to think about it as it only serves to drive me crazy. It is not something I can change – so why fret about it? But, like all people, I have my days.

Today, all that disappeared. Our new home is centrally located in our new town. This means I can walk to stores which our former home did not allow for. Freedom!

As I set out to walk down the street to a store, I almost felt giddy. Dawn's birthday is in three days and I was going to buy her a present. As I wandered through the store, it was hard to stay focused on picking out that right gift. I'm sure I must have been grinning from ear to ear. Once completed, I left with my bag and headed across the street to buy us ice-coffees.

A few minutes later, I was opening Dawn's home-office door and handed her the ice-coffee. She looked at me in shock and then a huge smile spread across her face. I smiled back. It has been a long time since I have had the pleasure of doing this.

We took our treat to the deck where I excitedly told Dawn of my adventures. We laughed together and all was good. Dawn teared up when I tried to describe this incredible feeling of freedom and independence.

I can't begin to thank Dawn enough in living carpe diem with me. She had lived in our old city for 23 years. We left it so that we can live in a small town on Lake Huron. In doing so, I now have freedom to wander into the town's stores, go to a coffee bar, and sit on a bench looking out at the peaceful water.

There is no pill that could ever make me feel the way I do right now. Freedom is a powerful emotion.

Understanding Dementia – Education for Health Professionals

Date: Aug. 18th, 2014

In November 2013, in partnership with Murray Alzheimer Research and Education (MAREP), a group of individuals living with dementia and their care partners, came together to discuss the lack of both Ontario and Canadian dementia strategy plans. Conversations were guided using the philosophy "Nothing about Us without Us." The primary goals of the meeting were to educate, create, and document recommendations which will significantly enhance the lives of those living with dementia and their care partners.

When creating and modifying Canadian polices about dementia, organizations must work in partnership and include representation from the population of those living with dementia. Ten recommendations were developed by this group with the intention of underlying what is most important to those living with dementia.

Number six on this list of ten recommendations is:

"Expand staff training and education - at all levels (e.g., physicians/ specialists to personal support workers, CCAC case managers, etc.)"

The other day, I picked up a copy of a "Health Care Newspaper." On one of its pages was a description of a full-day course titled "Understanding Dementia." Of course, this piqued my interest, and I reviewed its content.

In a former life, I was a Corporate Trainer which gives me a good understanding about course development and learning objectives. I was shocked to see how many topics this course was to cover. In fact, there were 25 in all. I figured it allocated on average about 15 minutes per topic. They are not small topics but rather large ones that in no way can be properly covered in 15 minutes. Examples include: Brain Ageing and memory; Reversible dementias; Huntington's disease; and treatments for Alzheimer's disease.

I reminded myself that perhaps the intent of the course is just to highlight these topics and not to actually "understand" them as suggested by the title of the course. This led me to review its Learning Objectives. This is the part of the course description that states participants completing this course will be able to _____(fill in the blank). For this course, the learners will be able to "discuss", "define", "outline" and "identify" different things about dementia. Hmm.

Its target audience is RNs, RPSs, LPNs, Pharmacists, Dietitians, Psychologists, and Social Workers.

Trying not to get my knickers-in-a-knot, I tried to look at the benefits of this course for the target audience. It will give the learner a brushstroke of information about dementia; Perhaps as a beginning course with more to follow.

Ask yourself the following question: Would you want to be assisted by a professional who only this course as their base of had "understanding dementia." For me, the answer is no. The obvious second question is: "How much "understanding dementia" is enough for health professionals to assist those with dementia?" The answer will depend on the individual and their healthcare role.

Once it is identified how much is needed for the individual or the profession, a gap analysis would be in order. If "x" is needed and the individual has "y" how does the profession intend to fill this educational gap? And when will it be filled?

This brings me back to the larger problem which is the lack of a Canadian and Ontario dementia plan. It is my assumption that if we had such plans, there would be an educational component to it. Within this component it would define what is needed for each profession and what it currently has (gap analysis). It would further define how it will address this information gap and by what date. A cohesive training plan would then be generated encouraging knowledge sharing and standardization.

Currently, some organizations and professions have already begun this important process of teaching their staff more about dementia as it relates to their own job. For instance, Schlegel Villages, owner and operator of several long-term care and retirement villages in Ontario, has a program titled "LIVING in MY TODAY." Developed in partnership with MAREP's Jessica Luh, the program has trained its own diverse facilitators – people from housekeeping, nurses, PSWs, food services, etc. This cross-section of facilitators ensures the training material reflects the needs of those in training. Ultimately, the way employees live and work with residents who are living with dementia will be reshaped.

Without a national and provincial dementia strategy, which will contain an education component, organizations and professionals will continue to develop and train in a silo and courses such as "Understanding Dementia" will continue to be developed.

Let's go Canada! It's time to make dementia education for our health professionals a priority.

Back to School

Date: Sept. 1St 2014

Back to school. Yes, hard to believe but summer is gone. For many, tomorrow brings the beginning of another school year. New shoes have been bought and are waiting for tomorrow to be put on. If you are like me, you know those new shoes enable you to run so much faster! For parents, its time for the routine to be reintroduced with a smile on your face. For those with dementia, this may also be a good time for you to take a new course to better understand dementia.

Dementia Alliance International (DAI), is doing the unprecedented – offering classes for people with dementia – taught by people with dementia. Woohoo! Congratulations DAI for continuing to break through barriers and bust false myths that people with dementia cannot learn anymore. And heaven forbid someone with dementia can be a great teacher. Who better to learn from than the person who has the disease?

DAI "Master Classes" are offered over the internet and are free to attend. Here is the current schedule:

Sept 3, 2014	I've Just Been Diagnosed. What's Next?
Sept 10th, 2014	My Conversation with My Doctor
Sept. 17th, 2014	Advocacy and Speaking Out
Sept. 24th, 2014	My Conversation with My Family

The four Master Classes topics are at the core for living well with dementia. It will help not just those newly diagnosed but anyone with dementia. Follow this link to learn more and sign up for the classes. Space is limited, so don't delay.

DAI Board Members are the panellists guiding the classes through its learning objectives. These are individuals who are not just members of the local dementia scene but are at the forefront in international dementia advocacy. It includes retired medical doctors.

One of my favourite lines to say is: "You learn something new everyday." Here is your chance to learn from the best. Time to go back to school.

Waiting for the Results

Date: Sept. 10th 2014

Do you ever let your breath out, and then realize that you had been holding it for months? Yesterday, that's how I felt.

For the past two years, I have been complaining to any doctor who will listen, that I have muscle twitches in my legs, feet, arms, and hands. They are sporadic. Further to that, I get muscle cramping in my thighs, usually at night.

My specialist doctor from Baycrest Hospital, in Toronto, is the first one to pickup on this and investigate further into the matter. Two months ago, he scheduled several tests to be performed. Yesterday, we travelled to Canada's largest ALS (Lou Gehrig's) clinic at Sunnybrook Hospital.

Amyotrophic Lateral Sclerosis (ALS) is a motor neuron disease. This progressive, usually fatal, neuromuscular disorder is caused by the gradual degeneration of the motor nerve cells that control voluntary muscle movement. For the past two months, I have tried not to let my thoughts lead me down the path of: "What if I have it..."

The interesting thing about having probable Frontotemporal Dementia, is that I am less empathetic and don't really get too nervous about things. Yesterday, I was a bit nervous.

I was scheduled for two tests. The first test was a Nerve Conduction Study (NCS) conducted by a technician. This measured my nerves' ability to send impulses to muscles in different areas of my body. It can determine if I have nerve damage or certain muscle diseases. For a period of about 20 minutes, the technician applied different levels of conduction resulting in small to larger twitches. I was surprised at how unpleasant it was.

The second test – Electromyogram (EMG) was performed by my doctor. During it, he inserted a needle electrode through my skin into various muscles. He pushed the needle around to test the electrical activity of my muscles when they contracted and when they are at rest.

I was encouraged by him as he gave the countdown of muscles from seven on down. After each muscle, he confidently said "normal." Dawn and I looked at each other and began to smile.

This doctor has a wonderful bedside manner and kind eyes. With each completed muscle, he informed us that the test results of today, and earlier, point to me not having ALS. Thank-you, thank-you, thank-you.

He continued on stating what I did have is "benign fasciculation syndrome (BFS). This is a neurological disorder characterized by fasciculation (twitching) of various muscles in the body. The precise cause of BFS is unknown. He went on to explain that this is not something to worry about. If I wish to check-in with him in a year's time, I was welcome. I smiled as I told him, "I hope I am a face that you will never see again."

As Dawn and I walked out of the hospital, I let out a big sigh. I realized I had been holding my breath for a very long time while waiting for my results.

Approximately 15% of patients with FTD also develop motor neuron disease with ALS being the most common type. I feel so fortunate to have ducked this "bullet."

I am so thankful to add BFS to my medical list. I simply cannot imagine the pain and sorrow of being diagnosed with ALS.

The Face of Dementia?

Date: October 1st, 2014

Scenario 1:
A middle-aged woman is walking her dog. She stops to chat with her neighbours. After a few minutes, she gives a wave and continues to walk her dog home.

Scenario 2:
An elderly woman sits in a chair. She is starring off into space and has a vacant look in her eye.

Question:
Which scenario describes a person with dementia?

Answer:
Both. Scenario 2 is a much-used media and medical portrayal of someone with dementia in its final stages. Scenario 1 is a little used portrayal of someone with dementia. According to many, the person "looks fine" therefore, can't have dementia.

If you chose scenario 2 as your answer, you have fallen into the stereotypical trap portraying the face of dementia. By doing so, you have inadvertently continued to perpetuate "the old face."

For those of us with early-onset dementia (people younger than 65), we are constantly challenged by this incorrect portrayal. It is common to hear from our own doctors, "You don't look sick. You look fine."

On a good note, many individuals, groups and organizations are working to overcome this prejudice. Efforts are being made to redefine the face of dementia. Bravo! This work will take many years as there is much to overcome.

Being an optimist, I believed most organizations are trying to move this effort forward. It is much to my chagrin that I found this not to be the case. I recently spoke with a peer from my own country of Canada. She has younger-onset dementia. She was telling me her story of wanting to volunteer.

Unfortunately, she was turned down because the employee felt because of her young age and "normal" appearance, she would not generate the amount of donations needed.

Hmm.

This is a reminder that the word about the new face of dementia is not being heard nor embraced by all who are affected by dementia. This is a serious issue. As individuals, we pick up clues from the media and the medical profession about what it is like to live with dementia. It seems that we are still focused on presenting it as late stage. For us, that means my scenario 2 – an older woman looking off into the distant with a vacant look in her eyes.

It takes time and effort to erase prejudice. It is a cause that is worthwhile and doable.

For someone who is just diagnosed with dementia, the saying "I can live well with dementia" is much more plausible if they can immediately reference my scenario 1. They do not need to go home, get their affairs in order, and stop living life. This is last stage dementia. There is so much more to living after a diagnosis. It is up to us to help change peoples understanding of early-stage onset and dementia in general.

The next time someone talks to you about dementia, I ask that you remember my face – the face of dementia.

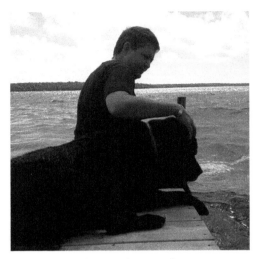

Shilo and me – The Face of Dementia

Lest We Forget

Date: November 8th, 2014

Last evening, Dawn and I enjoyed attending a local play titled "Homestead to War Front." The play recounted the young men who went off to the Great War, and how it affected the people left at home and the letters back and forth. The letters were actual correspondence from the war front to home.

During one scene, it dramatized two young men signing their Attestation papers. This scene hit home for me. I have a copy of my Grandfather, Fred Moran's, papers and of his brothers' Gordon Moran. On January 26th, 1915, Fred a 21-year-old unmarried sailor, answered the call to duty. As part of the 4th C.M.R. He did his best to defend his country. In the battle at Sanctuary Woods, he was shot in the stomach and laid in the mud for hours before medical attention could get to him. He was fortunate to survive and be part of another three years of battles in France.

They included Somme, Arras, Vimy Ridge, Hill 70, Kykpres, Passchendaele and Scarpe.

My grandfather was an extremely fortunate man in that he came home from this terrible Great war. He would latter marry my Grandmother and they would have five wonderful children.

His bother Gordon was not so lucky. On March 1916 this 18-year-old also answered the call of duty. He was able to survive the war but died from mustard gas poisoning in 1927 at d-Queen Alexandra sanatorium.

As the live theatre production continued, so did my reminiscing of other family members who were involved in WW1 and WWII.

My Grandpa Wighton listed at Essex county in Windsor, Ontario. At that time, he was already the father of three young boys. His friend encouraged him to enlist but stay in Canada. For most of the war he was stationed at the appropriated land of Stoney Point named Ipperwash camp, Ontario. It was a training camp. From 1942-1945 his duty was to help train bagpipers who then were sent overseas to the European theatre.

My Uncle Bill also was in WWII but as a Pathfinder Squadron, RCAF. The horrors of war never left him, and he spoke little about his experiences. He was fortunate and returned to his wife and young baby.

For my ancestors who lived in Scotland, they too experienced the horrors of war. Great Uncle William survived the war only to die later of Rheumatic fever which he acquired in the trenches of WW1.

His brother, Horace, who signed up when he was 21 was dead within the year. We can pay our respects to him in Alexandria War Cemetery, Egypt – Plot A 225.

More family names and faces appear on my list of "least we forget."

As Remembrance Day (Nov. 11th) approaches, I feel a change in Canadian attitude about honouring our men and women. This pass month, Canada has been under attack on our own soil. For over 150 years, this has not been the case. We have been blessed to live in a country where war and violence is not part of our culture. I am so proud of this fact. But now, due to the recent attacks, our military presence and strategy will/must change. Only time will tell how it will look.

For the many world war veterans who have dementia, I wonder if horrors of war were the first of memories to fade away. Or were they so horrific, they stayed with them.

For me, I have written down notes about my ancestors for me to remember. It will help me in remembering the many people around the world who have died in a war.

Lest we forget.

Humpty Dumpty

Date: November 29th, 2014

The last few weeks I have been "off." I have been extremely tired, lack motivation, and am moody. Today, I had another example of how my brain is changing.

I was tidying up the bedroom and began to move items in order to dust. I started to pile things on the dresser. I was not being careful but for some reason, didn't really care. As I continued, I looked at my South African art ostrich egg that was dangerously positioned underneath the piled-up items. I remember looking at it and thinking I should move it or else it will fall.

Well, guess what... it fell. Even though I had the initial thought of moving this precious piece of art, I didn't. I don't know why. All that I know is that the fragile Ostrich egg fell and shattered.

Dawn came running into the room and after surveying the floor she began to tear up. She knew how important this piece of art was to me. Several years ago, while working in South Africa, I bought this art Ostrich egg. It was the same day I went to Nelson Mandela's museum. I carefully carried it home and have always handled it with kid gloves. It meant a lot to me on an emotional level.

What is curious is what came to my brain next:

Humpty Dumpty sat on a wall; Humpty Dumpty had a great fall.

All the king's horses and all the king's men Couldn't put Humpty together again.

Strange. As I collected the pieces, it made me quite sad. But it was more than just a broken art piece. I felt sad because my brain did not do what it should have. One part of my brain should have said "danger, danger" this could fall and break. Another part of my brain should have then taken that piece of information and move the egg. It didn't.

As I looked down at the pieces, I thought to myself, this is like my brain. I now have these pieces that are disjointed and not connected anymore. So yes, the brain is still working, but not in the way it should; Much like Humpty Dumpty. It is quite a visual analogy for me.

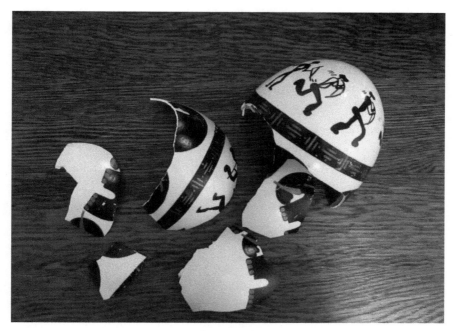

Broken Ostrich egg

As I lay contemplating this latest episode, I realize that just like Humpty Dumpty, I will not have someone who can fix me. Research and medical solutions are too far off in the future to be able to have the solution to glue those disjointed pieces of my brain back together.

With having dementia, I am very aware that I can present as looking fine. But my brain is sick and struggling. I will just have to continue to do my best and balance on the wall to the best of my ability.

Leon

Date: November 21st, 2014

Leon died last night. He is a man who I never had the pleasure to have met. But over the last year Dawn and I have learned about him and have grown to love him. He will be missed.

About one year ago, Dawn met Debbie, Leon's wife, through a web support group for people with Frontotemporal Lobe dementia (FTD). The two quickly became great friends and supports for each other.

They can relate to each other like no others. Depending on the day, Dawn and Debbie can be laughing or crying as they attempt to help keep each other strong in a long-distance relationship. Debbie and Leon live in Idaho, USA and we are in Southampton, Canada.

Through their marathon conversations, Dawn learned about Debbie's love of her life. Leon became sick about 10 years ago and was diagnosed with FTD six years ago. For about the last year he has been staying in a special home designed for those with cognitive challenges.

Leon enjoyed being taken on car rides while he drank his can of Coke and chewed gum while he listened to the car radio. He smoked and sang to the songs as Debbie and Leon meandered the countryside.

Dawn just spoke with Debbie a few days ago. Leon was not sick but was falling back into some manic behaviours. We don't know what happened and we wait to hear more about this sad news.

Dawn and I are always aware that I have a terminal illness. We know that in time, this will happen to us. It is something we try not to dwell on and keep focused on the many wonderful things' life has to offer.

But today, we are filled with sorrow for our friend Debbie. She is in our hearts and prayers. I hate this disease.

Dementia in the Workplace

Date: December 12th 2014

Recently, I have read some interesting articles on Dementia in the Workplace. Dementia by itself is challenging enough. But then to introduce the workplace to it? Yikes!

It has given me an opportunity to reflect on my own experiences. In the year 2007, I was 41 years old and the Vice-President and co-owner of a recruitment firm specializing in engineers. Prior to that position, I spent 10 extraordinarily successful years in the dot com business. I travelled the world, was a leader within my company, and managed hugely successful international teams and projects.

Somewhere along the way, I started to experience cognitive changes.

As the world economy spiralled down into a recession, the challenges to run a successful company became even that much more difficult. Eventually, the stress from it would culminate into a deep depression and I was ultimately put on leave by my doctor. The signs of dementia were already there, but my doctor looked for other diagnoses to explain these symptoms. How could I be 41 years old and have dementia?

Hindsight is a wonderful thing. For me, this is when I can reflect on the presence of symptoms of dementia while I was working.

But before I do that, let me remind you of the definition of dementia: "Dementia is a general term for a decline in mental ability severe enough to interfere with daily life."

While symptoms of dementia can vary greatly, at least two of the following core mental functions must be significantly impaired to be considered dementia:

- Memory
- Communication and language
- Ability to focus and pay attention
- Reasoning and judgment
- Visual perception
- People with dementia may have problems with short-term memory, keeping track of a purse or wallet, paying bills,

planning, and preparing meals, remembering appointments, or traveling out of the neighborhood."

Of the five core mental functions, all but visual perception affected me.

The issues were numerous and serious, considering my position. As VP, I was challenged at making executive decisions. I struggled with remembering employee results and if they were hitting targets. As my memory failed me, I looked for ways to try and compensate. I wrote more reminders and used "stickies" on everything. Discussions with clients became more difficult as I was unable to remember important details and information. It showed.

I was becoming mentally exhausted as I tried to keep focused. This resulted in me taking naps at lunch-hour and sleeping more and more.

Reasoning and judgement. I think of all the dementia symptoms, they affected me the most and were the earliest. I was not able to truly comprehend the financial struggles of the company.

Simply put, I made very serious errors which ultimately affected my family's finances which we will never recover from.

My emotions were hard to contain, and I lost control of my temper various times. I acted in an unprofessional manner and began to alienate my staff from me.

This subtle cognitive decline contributed to my deterioration to perform usual activities of daily living. Imagine if you had such symptoms. Would you be able to continue successfully with your job?

My family doctor put me on a medical leave from work. I have never returned.

Dementia in the workplace is a topic which demands more attention. Employees are retiring at an older age and due in part to improvements on diagnosing earlier, early-onset (beginning before the age of 65) dementia will become more prevalent. For those working with early-onset dementia, legally they must be protected. As always, education for both the employee and employer is crucial.

Learn the signs of dementia and never assume you are too young to have it. Just look at me.

The Spirit of Christmas

Date: Dec. 22 2014

When I was young, my favourite Christmas gift to open was always my stocking. Each of us 8 kids made our own stocking so there was quite a variety on how they looked. We always started with opening our stocking first. We could be sure to find an orange in the toe of it. This is a symbol for St. Nicholas.

It also contained some candy and other small toys. Today, I still love opening my stocking first to find out what treats are inside. Those small thoughtful gifts set the tone of the day for me. It is one of giving and special presents.

My other enduring memory of Christmas pass is of attending midnight mass. The hustle and bustle of the weeks preceding Dec.25th seemed to dissipate as the holy hour came upon us. Jamie O'Riley would sing from the choir, "O Holy Night." As I became swept up in the music it made me focus less on St. Nicholas and more on the Baby Jesus. His beautiful voice reminded me to acknowledge my blessed life.

We choose how the spirit of Christmas will be reflected. Is it all about presents, or does Jesus enter the picture as well? Put on some beautiful music like Jesu Joy of Man's Desiring, and let your heart be swept away. Then reach out to someone who may not be as blessed as you. Isn't that what Christmas is all about?

Merry Christmas Everyone!

YEAR FOUR

Put Your Money Where Your Mouth Is

Date: January 27th, 2015

It is hard to believe that the month of January nears its end as does Alzheimer Month Awareness. Canadians have been the target of multi- media campaigns focused to educate us on Alzheimer's and other dementias. There have been many inspiring and successful events including TV. Interviews, newsprint articles, internet media feeds, and of course The Walks.

Congratulations to the many people with dementia who have stood up and participated in the awareness – in whatever the capacity. And many thanks to all who have supported us in helping make these campaigns a success.

Once upon a time, I used to be a Project Manager of very large international projects. On completion of the projects, the team would come together and evaluate its success. We would reiterate our goals and then compare them to our results. The point of the exercise was to grow, learn from our mistakes, and celebrate our success. This was not always a fun way to spend a day at work. Sometimes, it was painful, and it was clear we could have done things differently for better results.

Why do I share this with you? My Project Manager instinct is bristling. I am pleased about the many successes of this month. Yet, during it I had an experience which has truly bothered me.

I was approached by an organization who wished to have me interviewed which would then be distributed via media outlets. I was happy to oblige, and the interview was published.

Initially, I thought it was a good interview. But something was bothering me about it. After a few days of mulling it over, I realized that it was a doom and gloom article. It stated the lead up to diagnosis and all the rotten symptoms which goes with having dementia. What it didn't say is I am living well with dementia; nothing about my advocacy work; no mention of the publication of my journals to international websites; missed the part stating I am part of a team working with the Ontario government in developing a Dementia Strategy to be implemented in the next 3-4 years.

Hmm. I asked myself why this article would be allowed to be published as it was negative and lacked inspiration. The article reaffirms the stigma which it is supposed to help fight against.

The Project Manager in me thought it was best to help identify to the Management Person the flaw in my interview. It did not meet the goals of the campaign.

I determined it was best for me to write an email to the Management Person. In it, I pointed out the good things but also made it clear that important information was not included. I also stated: "I truly believe it is vital that the stigma of the negative aspects of dementia need to be challenged and for people to understand and ultimately believe that there is life after diagnosis."

If a national campaign promotes a negative perspective, then others will follow.

It has now been two weeks since I emailed my suggestions to the Management Person. Much to my chagrin, it has not even been acknowledged. I ponder why this is so. I sent a copy of it to a colleague who gave me the thumbs up that it was professional in content.

How can a media campaign improve if its own Management Person is not willing to listen to feedback? If I were a person who didn't have dementia, would my email have been answered?

It seems that not everyone is truly working to reduce stigma and exclusion for those of us with dementia. It's time for all organizations to put their money where their mouth is.

Ontario Dementia Advisory Group

Date: February 25th, 2015

When I first started my journey of advocacy for those of us with dementia, I had no idea where it would lead to. I had little knowledge about the disease and the lack of government plans to help people with dementia live well with it. In other words, I was not aware that neither Canada nor Ontario had a Dementia Plan.

It did not take long, after my diagnosis, to determine I need to help others provide focus to this lack of clarity and initiative by the governments. Many people I have met, have spent literately years, trying to fight stigma, educate, and push for an Ontario Dementia Plan.

Those who have fought much longer than I, can be very proud that our day has finally come. Yes, Ontario is finally working towards a concrete Dementia Plan. It will take about four years from start to implementation.

In early December 2014, five people with dementia including myself, formed a group called Ontario Dementia Advisory Group. Included with us is our "support systems" people who help in enabling us to represent ourselves in a manner we wish to.

On February 4th, a historical meeting was held at the Niagara Alzheimer Society. In attendance was Ms. Indira Naidoo-Harris, MPP for Halton and Parliamentary Assistant to the Minister of Health and Long-Term Care, Dr. Eric Hoskins, and members of the newly developed Ontario Dementia Advisory Group (ODAG) and their support systems.

With great passion, ODAG members introduced Ms. Naidoo-Harris to two critically important documents developed by people with dementia:

1. "Engagement and Involvement in Public Policy", and

2. "Canadian National and Ontario Dementia Plans – Input from those living with Dementia."

The documents were received quite well, and with great emotion Ms. Naidoo-Harris vowed to ensure people living with dementia will be at the center of the newly forming Ontario Dementia Plan, which is her mandate.

I have included in this journal the document "Engagement and Involvement in Public Policy." I'm honoured to be a part of this group. I look forward to more accomplishments.

The words of Martin Luther King, ring in my ears: "Change does not roll in on the wheels of inevitability but comes through continuous struggle."

Engagement and Involvement in Public Policy

Dated: February 18, 2015
Forward

As a group of Ontarians living with dementia who are interested in being involved in public policy that will affect people living with dementia across Ontario, we have developed this document to provide an outline of what we feel it means to be engaged in public policy activities. We believe this will help with understanding the best manner of moving forward in any new partnerships and will assist all stakeholders involved in this process.

It is also important to note, that our care partners have their own perspectives which should be listened to. This can be done separately from our own involvement. By having two distinct meetings, we ensure our views are heard and not overwhelmed by our care partners.

Furthermore, collective engagement is a powerful alternative to meetings with individuals. Being in a group setting provides opportunities for each member of the group to contribute and help others in their contributions if needed. This makes us stronger and more unified in our quest for "nothing about us without us."

The information presented in this document is a summary of discussions our group has had and informed by the work conducted by:

Dementia North, UK - Listen to Us: Involving people with dementia in planning and developing services

Meaningful Engagement Framework developed Wiersma et al., (2014)

The Authentic Partnership Approach developed by MAREP

National Older Person's Mental Health Program, UK – Strengthening the Involvement of People with Dementia: A Resource for Implementation

As people living with dementia, we have personal perspectives about dementia that no one else has. We recognize that the involvement of people living with dementia has lagged other groups because there are often assumptions that people living with dementia are unable to communicate their needs, wants, and perspectives with others. This has led to social exclusion, and this is something we find unacceptable.

We are still the same people we were prior to our diagnosis. We have a lifetime of knowledge and experience to share. Life does not end when you receive that diagnosis, and we want to reinforce that each person living with dementia is still a whole person with much to contribute. When provided the opportunity to have our voices heard, we can communicate how dementia affects us and how services should meet our health and social needs.

Involvement versus Consultation

We believe there is an important distinction between involvement of people living with dementia and consulting people living with dementia.

Consultation tends to be a one-off event, which includes focus groups or questionnaires to receive feedback from stakeholders. This type of approach is helpful in specific circumstances, but it lacks the commitment of meaningful continued involvement in the process of decision-making.

Involvement is a process and not a one -off event. To really engage and involve people living with dementia, a commitment to greater involvement needs to be explicit and planned.

What is Engagement?

Engagement refers to the way you involve people living with dementia throughout the process of developing, implementing, and evaluating policy.

This process should be conducted in a culturally sensitive manner.

The following points should be kept in mind when engaging with people living with dementia:

- Recognize the expertise that people living with dementia bring to decision-making and that we should be considered key stakeholders, not an afterthought.
- Recognize that power imbalances exist between people living with dementia, care partners, service providers and other stakeholders, and work to provide equal footing.
- Look to develop a partnership rather than one-off consultations and provide consistent updates as the project moves forward.
- Be open to adapting your practices based on feedback received from people with dementia during the process of engagement.
- Value personhood based on a holistic appreciation of the emotional, social, spiritual and artistic dimensions of individuals.
- Each person's experience of dementia is unique, but there are certain realities that need to be remembered as you move to involve people with dementia in public policy work.
- Engagement is an exhausting process for all involved. There needs to be recognition that on some days, people will be better at contributing than other days, just like with anyone.
- The appropriateness of approaches, activities, and methods needs to be considered in relation to the abilities and characteristics of the people living with dementia being engaged.
- Recognize the value of the collective engagement experience: Engaging with others as a group allows us to support each other to overcome some common challenges, such as:
- Difficulty concentrating
- Memory lapses
- Difficulty retrieving information

- Time to absorb information

Translate into action the views and experiences gathered through involvement.

To overcome the imbalances in power between people living with dementia, care partners and service providers, it's important to ask "what degree of control and influence do people living with dementia really have? How does it compare to care partners? How does this compare to other stakeholders?"

Below is a list of practical considerations that need to be made when facilitating the engagement process (Borrowed from "Listen to Us: Involving people with dementia in planning and developing services" developed by Dementia North in the UK).

Facilitating the process:

- Do not assume that the issues identified for consultation are important issues for the people with dementia. Ask them for their agendas.
- At each meeting, spend some time prompting and reminding the people with dementia who you are and what you discussed at the previous meeting.
- Take time to talk – don't be hurried.
- Allow for periods of silence to assist with absorbing information.
- Do not try to move people on at a faster pace than they are able to cope with.
- Recognise that the views of the person with dementia may change in the course of a meeting or from day to day, as well as over longer periods.
- Ensure that options and the implications of any choices made by an individual or the group are understood.
- Check that the participants agree with any views or suggestions recorded.
- When people with dementia are participating in formal meetings, ensure that minutes and other documents are delivered to

them well before the meeting to allow them time to consider the content and to prepare to present their views. Ask them when they would prefer to receive these documents. Aid with this if required.

- Arrange for people with dementia who are participating in formal meetings to be supported, as required, to present their views.

Summary

- Focus on what we can do, not on what we can't do.
- Acknowledge the power of collective engagement in enhancing our ability to overcome challenges.
- Life doesn't stop when you receive a diagnosis. Our ability to access this information may change, but our personal histories and experiences are still there.
- We are more than our diagnosis.

* * *

Members
Bea Kraayenhof, Welland
Bill Heibein, Thunder Bay
Brenda Hounam, Paris
Maisie Jackson, Niagara Falls
Mary Beth Wighton, Southampton, Bruce County

Partners
Alzheimer Society of Ontario: Delia Sinclair Frigault, Phil Caffery, Nancy Rushford
Alzheimer Society of Niagara Region: Gina Bendo
Centre for Education and Research on Aging & Health (CERAH) at Lakehead University: Elaine Wiersma
Murray Alzheimer Research and Education Program (MAREP) at the University of Waterloo: Lisa Loiselle

Musing about "Still Alice"

Date: March 2nd 2015

There has been a great deal of discussion surrounding the recently released movie "Still Alice." Actress Julian Moore, who portrays Dr. Alice Howland, has won the coveted Academy Award for Best Actress. The movie is about a renowned linguistics professor. Words begin to escape her, and her memory begins to fail her. She is diagnosed with early-onset Alzheimer's disease. From her first-hand narrative perspective, we go through her struggles and fears with her.

I have been asked several times if I have watched this movie. No, I haven't it. But, when I was first diagnosed with probable Frontemporal Dementia (FTD), the book, written by Lisa Genova, was given to me. As a book, it rates high on the list of "must reads" along with the "The 36-Hour Day." The first support people we met with suggested reading it along with other material.

I took everyone's advice and read the book. I shouldn't have – at least not that early in my diagnosis. When I was first diagnosed, I was reading everything I could to better understand this disease. For the most part, the reading material was quite factual, or it was from the perspective of a care support person. It most definitely was not from the perspective of the person with dementia which is the kind of narrative used in "Still Alice."

I remember when I finished reading the last page, I felt strangely uncomfortable. This story had taken me on a journey which included making plans for suicide when the disease threatened to overtake Alice. I was frightened by story.

For me, the book was not just a story, but rather a possible journey which I would take as I too had dementia. I wondered to myself if I would do those things – or didn't do those things – that Alice did. Would I get lost 3 blocks from my house? Would I forget the month? Or birthday of my spouse? When would I start to place my cell phone in crazy places like the microwave? Would my world become lonely like Alice's'?

Since several people had wondered about my opinion of the movie, I decided to reread the book again. Maybe I would have a different take on it. I have.

When I picked up the book to reread it, the first thing I did was to read The Acknowledgments. I don't remember if I did it the first time. But this time I recognized a list of who's-who of advocates who have dementia. In fact, I have been in correspondence or on conference calls with some of them. Genova has certainly used the best experts to help in her story telling.

Today, I received a report from my Baycrest doctor. It explains my cognitive challenges and language difficulties. So, when today I read the paragraph in the book about "word finding" I instantly related to it. She simply couldn't find the word. She had a loose sense for what she wanted to say, but the word itself eluded her. Gone. She didn't know the first letter or what the word sounded like or how many syllables it had. It wasn't on the tip of her tongue."

While I was rereading the book, I discovered similarities to Alice, that I did not have before. One of my biggest changes is in my diet and the liking of certain foods. My food preferences have changed considerably. I prefer cereal (usually a granola kind), over any other type of food. I will tell Dawn, "I don't like that" when I'm told I used to like it. Texture and smells will easily put me off and I will simply refuse to eat what is placed in front of me.

It made me smile, therefore, when I read the scene about Alice asking for coffee and her husband stating, "You don't like coffee." And then the back and forth about her like or dislike for coffee. Once again, this rang true to me.

It still pains me to read any articles, including "Still Alice" about the description of its final stages of the disease: "She'd be unable to feed herself, unable to talk, unable to recognize John and her children. She'd be curled up in the fetal position, and because she'd forget how to swallow, she'd develop pneumonia."

Dawn and I have had many conversations about the practicality of me living in our home if possible. We have also toured different long-term care facilities and reviewed the cost of living in a home. Once again, Alice goes through the same motions. She visits a dementia ward and is told the rate runs at $285/day. And like Alice, Dawn and I can no longer imagine me in a dementia ward as we can shelling out a lot of money to live in it.

Alice also wishes she had any other disease. Especially a disease in which people can see that you are sick. With dementia, especially for young onset, many times we are told "you look fine." I know exactly what Alice is thinking about.

This time, when I read "Still Alice" I decided to bookmark pages in which there was similarity. I wanted to see if I related better to Alice than I did two years ago. When I turned to the last page, I had more book-marks than I could easily count. I have changed – just like Alice.

I ask myself if I would recommend this book to someone newly diagnosed. I don't believe I would. The story of Alice is about a woman checking periodically that she can perform certain things. And if she can't, then in her eyes she is no longer herself – Alice. It is then she should take several pills and fall asleep forever.

For someone newly diagnosed, we are told and given materials which explains dementia. To read a book about someone wanting to commit suicide was too much for me. It took my heart to a place I was not prepared to go.

What would I suggest? Hmm. I'm not sure it is written yet. But I would want it to take me on an open and honest journey. But perhaps, give more weight to the fact that you can still live well with dementia.

Mom

Date: March 18, 2015

It was 10 days ago, when I stood with my family and prayed over my Mom's coffin.

The words of the priest were lost on me as my mind was saturated with memories and my heart of sorrow. Mom died at 87 years old of Alzheimer's disease.

When I reflect on these past three weeks, it is a blur.

I am so thankful for being able to spend the night with her before her passing. I was able to sit beside her and whisper my love to her. I played our favourite songs and told her funny stories. I touched her cheek, held her hand and ran my hand through her silky white hair.

I cherish that night. It was beautiful, peaceful evening. Although she slept during it, I know her spirit was there with me.

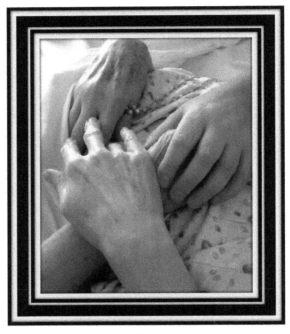

Hands

She would have been immensely proud of her family as we pulled together and utilized all our individual talents and gave her a beautiful mass with many of us contributing in some small way. The church was full of the many people whose lives my Mom had touched. We have an exceptionally large family. She was the Mother of eight children and their spouses, and had 20 grandchildren, and 14 great-grandchildren.

I am so fortunate to be part of a loving family who worked hard to ensure Mom lived well with dementia. We supported Dad who never could comprehend how his wife of 64 years couldn't remember a holiday they took.

I know it is because of my family, that Mom's quality of life was enriched because of their direct and indirect actions. I am so thankful to them.

I miss my Mom. But I know she is with me in my heart and looks over me from heaven.

The Robin

Date: April 12, 2015

I have debated whether to write this journal. Reader, you may think I have lost my marbles. I can assure you I haven't. Perhaps the best way to start this is to declare "truth is stranger than fiction."

Five years ago, my brother Gregory died after a very brief battle with cancer. Shortly after this, I began to have strange encounters with Red Cardinals. They appeared on our back porch, other places where I had never seen them; and their black faces looked directly at me. It was as if the Red Cardinal was sending me messages to be strong and hold the faith. I just knew it was my brother Gregory somehow trying to give me strength in my own battle with dementia.

I have had this strange experience once again.

It has been just over a month since my Mom passed from Alzheimer's disease. Almost immediately, I noticed a Robin hopping around – as if it were trying to get my attention. This has happened numerous times this month.

Once, while we were out driving, a Red Cardinal flew directly across our path, followed by a Robin crossing in the other direction. Yes, it was uncanny.

Last night while taking my dog Shiloh out for a walk, I turned down a street that was quite short. Robins began to appear on either side of the road. They were hopping or flying along with us. I know, this sounds crazy.

It was so weird; I began to laugh out loud. Mom, through the beautiful Robin is sending me strength and courage.

As I look forward to the next few years, I believe I have a lot of advocacy work to complete. To help Ontario create and implement an Ontario Dementia Strategy. I have been feeling mentally exhausted and question my ability, courage, and strength to participate in such important work.

Mom was a humble person who took part in many organizations to help the less fortunate. This was important to her and she did it all her life. I learned the importance of advocacy from her.

Maybe that as dementia continues to fight for control of my brain, my other senses have become stronger. Perhaps this is how I can explain my experiences with The Robin. I'm more keenly aware of such possibilities.

But then, perhaps there isn't an explanation. It simply just is. It is The Robin.

Canada – Conservative's withdraw support for Bill-356 – National Dementia Strategy!

Date: April 22nd 2015

I shake my head in disappointment and in frustration.

Two days ago, Dawn was speaking with her good friend Matt Dineen whose 43-year-old wife is in long-term care with Frontotemporal dementia (FTD). Matt, a national supporter of Bill-356, spoke with Dawn about the Conservative government withdrawing their support for this bill – which is a National Dementia strategy. All other parties support this bill. On May 6th, there will be a vote. Unless members of the Conservative government vote with their conscious, it will not pass. Canada will be the only G7 country STILL to not to have a strategy.

My family was busy yesterday – writing to Conservative MP's and faxing letters pushing for MPs to support this bill.

Canadians – I plead to you that you also pick up your pen and write to the government pushing for support. Time is of the essence.

Below is the letter I sent. Feel free to copy parts of this letter that makes sense for you.

Dear Member of Parliament:

I am writing concerning the upcoming vote (May 6th) on Bill- 356, *An Act respecting a National Strategy for Dementia*. Despite your government's opposition to this bill, I appeal to you today to consider my own personal story, and to vote with your conscience, regardless of your party's position.

I am 48 years of age, a retired vice-president and owner of a recruiting firm. In addition, I spent 10 years in the dot com business as a Sr. Business Analyst. In September 2012, I was diagnosed with probable Frontotemporal Dementia (FTD), a debilitating disease for which there is no known cure (and a life expectancy of 7-13 years on average). My drivers license was immediately revoked, and I was instructed to "put my affair in order." Basically, I was informed I would no longer be useful to society nor can have a good life. My partner of 13 years, Dawn, and daughter Brianna have not accepted this prescription to death, but instead have adopted the motto "carpe diem." To that, I can say I am living well with dementia.

I am an advocate at all levels to fight stigma, educate about dementia, and look to partner with others so people with dementia can be the center of our own healthcare. The simple reason being we are the experts.

I am a strong supporter for a national dementia plan and support the private member's bill. It is concrete legislation that, if passed, will mandate action for a national plan.

I was shocked when your government on March 13 announced it would oppose bill C-356, introducing instead its own motion, that focuses more on research and public awareness. This non-binding motion rather than a law means no mandate to act, no real leadership from Ottawa, no help now for me, others with dementia, and for Dawn

– my care partner and other health care providers. How will this motion keep me at home for as long as possible?

It goes without saying that the issue of dementia should be non-partisan. I plead with you to vote with your conscience and do what you know is right and vote in favour of the private member bill on May 6th.

World FTD Awareness Week

Date: August 20th, 2015

I remember sitting next to the geriatrician as she looked at me and Dawn and said that I mostly like to have FTD or Frontotemporal dementia. It used to be called Pick's disease.

This sounded serious, so I listened more intently. She continued to inform us that there is no cure and on average life expectancy ranges from 2 – 8 years. The doctor continued to rattle on that due to my extensive amount of education (6.5 years of post-secondary) it will help in slowing things down. She explained that the disorder affects the frontal and temporal lobes of the brain and average onset age is 57. She also stated she had little experience with FTD and I was the youngest patient she had. She encouraged us to contact the Alzheimer Society as they were the "experts."

She announced that because FTD affects decision making, she was immediately revoking my license and I was no longer allowed to drive.

I stopped hearing. I could no longer absorb anything that she said. I looked at Dawn who had a "deer in the headlight" look.

I could feel years of frustration bubbling up. It had taken four years to get to this point. Years of being told I had depression, cognitive impairment, post-traumatic stress disorder, conversion disorder, etc. Now, I was told that I can't drive, and I will die from this disease that I knew nothing about.

Some words from the doctor floated into my brain: get your things in order; probably end up living in long-term care home; my drivers license was revoked.

I could not listen to her anymore. I stood up, threw some sheets of paper in the air, slammed the office door a few times and left the room. I paced in the hall and waited for Dawn to join me shortly. We drove home in silence – each lost in our own thoughts – and Dawn occupying my drivers' seat.

At home, at some point, I picked up the literature the doctor had given Dawn regarding the disease. There was one pamphlet and a few other information sheets from the Alzheimer Society. The doctor had written on the "Pick's" pamphlet the word "FTD."

Other than one other sheet, all documentation referred to Alzheimer's disease – which I do not have. Useless.

Over the next few days there were a flurry of telephone calls. As Dawn spoke to numerous people, I began to research this new word "frontotemporal dementia." I discovered there are three types:

1. Progressive behavior/personality decline—characterized by changes in personality, behavior, emotions, and judgment (called behavioral variant frontotemporal dementia)

2. Progressive language decline—marked by early changes in language ability, including speaking, understanding, reading, and writing (called primary progressive aphasia).

3. Progressive motor decline—characterized by various difficulties with physical movement, including the use of one or more limbs, shaking, difficulty walking, frequent falls, and poor coordination (called corticobasal syndrome, supranuclear palsy, or amyotrophic lateral sclerosis).

I then realized the doctor had not defined which type I had – only that I had probable FTD. As I looked through the symptoms of each, I knew that I most likely had behavioural variant frontotemporal dementia (bvFTD).

When Dawn and I regrouped and she shared what she had learned and I the same, we quickly realized that few people knew very much about bvFTD. Most of the documentation we received was regarding

Alzheimer's disease. Something I don't have. Also, my young age of 46 proved a challenge as most programs were geared for the elderly.

We felt very alone with few options and we were very worried.

During this period, Dawn met Matt Dineen through a support group. Matt's wife, Lisa, has bvFTD and is living in a long-term care facility. She is 44 years old. Matt and Dawn quickly became friends and confidantes. We learned that Matt is an activist for FTD and other dementias. He is well-known in the Canadian political world as he is constantly contacting MPPs and other dignitaries to push for further education, support, and aid for those with FTD. I am proud to call Matt my friend.

Recently, Matt and others of like mind, have accomplished an extraordinary thing of organizing for the first time, countries across the globe who will observe World FTD Awareness Week from October 4th – October 11th, 2015. At least 10 countries will collaborate on many exciting events and outreach activities. The City of Ottawa has already embraced this and had proclaimed this as World FTD Awareness Week in Ottawa. The shared aim is to ensure awareness and improve access to support wherever there are families impacted by FTD, while fostering research that will lead to a cure.

FTD accounts for nearly 5% of all 750,000 dementia cases in Canada. That means I am one of 37,500 people in this special group that I would rather not be a part of.

There are many other types of dementia's other than just Alzheimer's, which traditionally receives the most attention and funding. There is FTD which few people know about including those in the health care sector.

I urge you to assist in helping those of us with FTD by joining in the week of Oct 4-11th 2015. Thank you for taking the time to understand my disease better. Dawn and I never want anyone else to go through what we have... what we are...and what we will.

Canadian Parliament votes NO for National Strategy for Dementia

Date: May 7th, 2015

Yesterday, Canadian Parliament decided the course for years to come for dementia in Canada. In a nail-biting vote it was decided by 139 to 140 <u>against</u> Bill C-356 – An Act Respecting a National Strategy for Dementia.

My family has licked envelopes, faxed, emailed, and talked with many members of parliament to encourage them to vote "Yeah" for the Bill. The Ontario Dementia Advisory Group, of which I am a member, has emailed all Ontario Conservative MP's pleading with them that they vote "Yeah" for the Bill and against party politics. Other individuals, groups, committees, and Church organizations have also been working extremely hard to educate the public on this Bill and the impact on them if it is passed.

As someone with dementia, I have racked my brain trying to come up with various strategies to reach out to all who will listen on what **I** need – which is this Bill.

I applaud all individual Members of Parliament who voted for it. I'm sure their constituency is happy with them.

Considering the subject, it is shameful to report that this was a political party vote.

I am even more perplexed to discover that the of Minister of Health, voted Nay to Bill C-356.

I'm not a politician. I'm simply a 48-year-old woman who is living well with probable Frontotemporal dementia. I do not understand the "things behind the scenes" which comprises politics. I'm simply a person with dementia trying to understand why my government has chosen to

limp along with a health care system that has piece-meal solutions for a dementia strategy. I'm simply a person living with dementia who is worried how my family and myself will overcome the many hurdles in our way because of the lack of enough well-educated health staff, research, funding and leadership. I'm simply a person with dementia working with other persons with dementia who want to be the center of our own healthcare and are working hard to have our voices heard above all political bullshit. I'm simply a person with dementia who can't explain to people with dementia in other G8 countries why Canada's Minister of Health, despite all evidence provided to her, voted Nay.

Perhaps the answer I try to understand is as simple as that. It's party politics.

As the old saying goes, "They have won the fight, but they haven't won the war." We will keep on fighting for what makes sense: A national strategy for dementia.

Tough Advocate Decision

Date: May 18, 2015

When I was little, and someone asked me what I wanted to be when I grew up, "advocate" was not among my list. I was leaning more towards a teacher or a pro basketball player. But life doesn't always go the way you think it is going to. And so here I am today – an advocate.

Merriam-Webster dictionary defines advocate as: "a person who argues for or supports a cause or policy." I remember in the introduction of my first public speech, I was referred to as an advocate. It made me pause and wonder.... is that what I am now? It also made me feel a sense of pride and important.

I threw myself 110% into my new occupation. There was so much to learn and so much to do. I joined groups, helped with projects, and always sought to educate others about dementia. I was quite happy with dementia consuming my life.

Lately, I have begun to question my advocacy role. I do not spend anywhere near the time I used to fight for the cause. There are a few reasons for this: I no longer live in a large city with many advocacy projects available; I have spent more time with my favorite hobbies including finding new ones; I am frustrated by the repeated failings of advocacy projects in the world including my own back yard, and I enjoy other past-times.

How much time and work do you need to do until you are an advocate? I like this vocation calling and would hate to lose it.

Yesterday, Dawn and I lived carpe diem at its best. We did not have a set agenda for the day, so lived by impulse. For a while we sat by the pond feeding the ducks. It was busier than normal with vacationers. The kids oohed and ahhed at the large carpe as they came up in the water. It was easy and enjoyable.

We took a drive along Lake Huron and absorbed the beauty and admired the well- kept homes over looking the lake. We had an ice cream cone and homemade hamburgers. I sat on our deck and watched the birds jockey for position on the bird feeder to enjoy their new striped sunflower feed. As the day came to an end, I fished off the dock – never caring if I caught a fish. The sky became a million-dollar canvas with an incredible sunset. Life could not be any grander.

We also did more thing – we looked at a new rental home that has a two-minute walk to either the river or the lake. Our one-year commitment in this rental is coming quickly to a close and we do not wish to renew it. By the end of May we need to decide if we are moving back home to the city. We have rented it out for one year. We know our tenant loves our home and wants to still rent from us. That's not the issue. The issue is do we go back or not.

As we keep reviewing our list of pros and cons, I find myself stumped by how much time do I wish to allocate to advocacy work. It is easier to do this in the city as there are more opportunities for it, and I would be right in the room with others. Not so for Southampton. I'm far enough way to even make it difficult for me to be interviewed by media. Their only solution is telephone and that means I miss out on media opportunities. Yes, I can use technology and that most certainly helps – but its not the same. When using technology, someone with dementia can easily miss nuisances and important pieces of information. It usually is harder to follow.

I have a tough decision in front of me. My involvement with being a dementia advocate is important and rewarding work. But, is it more rewarding than living carpe diem with my Dawnie Girl?

Reader, I don't know the answer. I'll let you know in two weeks.

What Would Batman Do?

Date: June 2nd 2015

I was born in 1966 which is the same year the TV series "Batman" debuted. When I was a bit older, I used to love watching the Caped Crusader battle evil- doers in Gotham city. I was enthralled by the words "BOOM", "BANG", "ZAP" splattered across the TV screen. My friends and I would run through the park singing at the top of our lungs, the upbeat title song: "NA NA NA NA NA NA NA NA Batman..." It was a time of innocence in which it was clear who was the good guy and who was the villain.

Fast forward to today. As of late my journals have taken on a political tone. I realize that to be an effect advocate I must be knowledgeable of the political world concerning dementia. I have read and spoken with people about bills, motions, and strategies so I better understand where the hold up is regarding people living with dementia to live better. It saddens me to now know that so much of it hinges on political gain.

Yesterday, I became inspired by that old Batman title song. The fight of good versus bad can be applied to the politics of dementia. I wonder what Batman would do to convince the politicians that a national dementia strategy is needed?

Why Do You Not Believe Me?

Date: July 2nd 2015

When I say I have dementia, there is usually a stigmatized response: "Gee you don't look sick." "You are too young to have dementia." "I'm not good at math either." "Everyone gets forgetful."

What I find surprising is that some of these stigmatized responses come from people who know me, have direct contact with me and are recipients of my advocacy work. It is as if they don't believe I have a disease that has no cure and ultimately will die from. One such person said that I "...can walk and talk so *I'm fine*."

What else do I need to do for <u>all</u> people to believe me? Perhaps the better question is why do I feel the need to convince them? And why am I disappointed, hurt and sometimes angry with them that they don't? Rest assured I have received a diagnosis of probable Frontemporal dementia. I have been through the gamete in seeing doctors, tests, and been under high scrutiny. My brain has been picked and prodded at.

I'm so sick of it, that I have told Dawn I'm done with doctors and don't want to see and more. I will do the basic requirements necessary for me to retain my personal insurance. That most likely means a yearly visit to the world-renowned brain hospital Baycrest to see the Head, Division of Neurology.

I'm reminded of the apostle "Doubting Thomas" who refused to believe that the resurrected Jesus had appeared to the other apostles until he could see and feel the wounds of Jesus. Skeptic, why do you not believe I have dementia? I am unable to show you my diseased neurons that are not firing on all cylinders.

I am not alone in this as most people having dementia experience this stigma. I am fortunate in that I have an early diagnosis. This has enabled me to have the time and ability to learn about my diagnosis and prepare accordingly.

Dementia does not mean I am old and always forgetful.

Skeptic, I:

- am a person
- have a diagnosis of dementia
- have great long-term memory
- struggle with short-term memory
- struggle with making decisions
- struggle with math
- struggle with understanding humour
- struggle with understanding complex movies
- struggle with word finding
- am not as compassionate to others as I once was,
- take a great deal of medication that makes me tired (not lazy), and
- I am loved by many.

Reader take the time to understand dementia. It doesn't take long. Educate yourself.

I would hate to think that you too are a skeptic.

Nightmares or the Orange Pill

Date: July 15 2015

I'm tired this morning. The lingering effects of my nightmares stays with me.

One of the characteristics of Frontotemporal dementia is sleep disturbances. In addition to this I have been diagnosed with REM sleep behavioural disorder. This "… is a disorder in which you physically act out vivid, often unpleasant dreams with vocal sounds and sudden, often violent arm and leg movements during REM sleep."

Normally you don't move during REM sleep. About 20 % of your sleep is spent in REM sleep, the usual time for dreaming, which occurs primarily during the second half of the night.

REM sleep behaviour disorder often may be associated with other neurological conditions such as Lewy body dementia, Parkinson's disease, or multiple system atrophy.

I have had this disorder for about four years; That means prior to my diagnosis of Frontemporal dementia (FTD). The other distinct characteristic of this is that you usually remember the nightmare(s) unlike many dreams.

Although I had a diagnosis, I choose not to take any suggested medications to help the symptoms. About a year ago, that changed as my nightmares were more frequent and frightening. My doctor put me on 0.5MG of Clonazepam. Yes, medication from the "pam family." Clonazepam often used to treat anxiety is also the traditional choice for treating REM sleep behaviour disorder.

However, in people with FTD, benzodiazepines have been associated with an increase in behavioural challenges and impair both memory and psychomotor skills. Use can result in reduced inhibition and impaired judgement. Simply put Clonazepam should be avoided.

I'm sure you can see the conundrum. To take or not to take. That is the question!

My daily medication is taken via a blister-pack. The clonazepam is not included in it. Every night as I take my blister-pack medication, I must also open the pill bottle for it.

Last night I choose not to take it. This is the second time this week. Why not? I keep hoping to take less medication. I keep thinking maybe I don't need to take it anymore. But I'm promptly reminded why I do need to take it. Without it comes the nightmares. Terrible nightmares.

Although clonazepam is not suggested for people with dementia, I've made a choice to include the orange pill in my daily medication. Without it, the monsters come out and I can be heard yelling "Help me...."

My Friend Carl Wilson

Date: July 8th, 2015

If you are extremely fortunate, you will meet a person in your life who will have a profound impact on you. January 23rd, 2013, I met this person. His name: Carl Wilson.

I was one of three speakers at a University of Waterloo forum on Alzheimer's disease presented by MAREP. It was my first public appearances, and I was nervous. I was the last speaker and Ann Marie Wilson, Carls' wife, spoke before me.

Anne Marie shared the story of Carl who was maintaining a healthy and a purposeful life despite Alzheimer's. Carl sat in the front row and encouraged his wife through claps and tears of joy. He smiled non-stop. I was immediately taken to him.

During my speech, Carl was intently listening and encouraged me as well through his purposeful communication methods. I felt stronger and less nervous. At the end of it, I knew I had made him proud by his tears of joy. I have never forgotten this.

Though the local advocacy grapevine, I would hear of the amazing work this wonderful couple were involved in. At once such event, a local T.V. Interview, we both were so excited to see each other. I sat beside him, and we held hands smiling and laughing. I tapped into his electric energy to help charge my battery.

The last time I saw Carl was at an Alzheimer's Walk. He had his family surrounding him and the crowd cheered on this iconic image. We once again clasped hands and smiled and laughed. It felt wonderful to be in his presence.

Every so often, Ann Marie emails me with the latest news about Carl. Ann Marie ensured that Carl lived the best he could with dignity and love. From her emails, I knew Carl was declining.

Today, Ann Marie sent me an email. Carl died peacefully this past Saturday. My heart hurts for Ann Marie and her family. They will miss Carl tremendously.

It is hard to describe the impact this has had on me. The reality is, Carl and I only met a few times and spent a bit of time with each other. But I felt this magnetic draw to him. Although challenged to verbally communicate, he was able to strongly affect me by other methods of communication. It must have been wonderful to have this man as a husband, father, friend, etc.

I am fortunate to have met Carl and Ann Marie. They have showed be the strength of a loving couple and that you can still have a great life regardless of Alzheimer's.

In the future, when I am speaking at events, I will imagine Carl sitting in the front row cheering me on. Thank you, my friend, – rest in peace.

Breaking the Law

Date: July 24, 2015

I have been a law-abiding citizen for all my life – well, give or take a speeding ticket. I respect police officers and appreciate their work in helping to keep our streets safe.

Therefore, it was a strange experience to be sitting in the front seat of our car being questioned by a policeman about my recent disturbance in a computer store. It never was supposed to happen like it did.

It all started several weeks ago when I began to have trouble with my new computer dropping my WiFi network. I could only work in one room and if I left it, the network dropped, and I couldn't access the internet. This was a big issue for me.

We had the internet company come out three times to check our router and ensure it was working properly – which it was. The next step was to take it back to our local computer store where we bought the computer. The store owner servicing me lacked professionalism and it annoyed me how he spoke down to me. He talked me into buying a software package which "most likely" will fix the problem. It didn't and I now was in the hole for $75.

I took my computer back to the store for the second time and spoke with the same man. He took the computer for the day to work on it. Once again, we picked it up only for it to still not work. We returned a third time where he said the entire computer needed to be sent back to the manufacturer as it had a faulty network card. It would take 7-10 business days to be fixed. He told me I would be called when it was done. By then, it was obvious we rubbed the owner the wrong way as he did with us. It was difficult to get what was needed for the computer to be fixed. By now I am aggravated.

I use my computer every day. It plays a big part in keeping me connected with others, informed, has my games on it and all my files. It was not easy to be without my computer for 10 days.

Yesterday, Dawn drove me to the store as I was told it was fixed when I called for an update. In the store I was told by the technician that nothing was wrong with it and it was never sent away. So, it had just been sitting there for 10 days.

Something clicked in my brain. I could see fire and my vision became focused on one person – the condescending owner. I marched up to him and told him he lied to me. It was to be sent away and for me to get a new network card. He just kept staring at me with this annoying look and repeatedly said, "My technician said there is nothing wrong with it."

I began to yell at him calling him a liar and that he needed to fix my computer which was still under warranty. He refused. I stood in the middle of the small store yelling when Dawn came in to see what was causing the delay. Instantly she understood the gravity of the situation and urged me to leave the store.

After some coxing, she led me out to our car where I sat for about one minute. I opened the door of our moving car and barged back into the store. He had been smirking and laughing at us. I couldn't stand it.

I don't know why I returned to the store. There was nothing positive to come of it. The first item closest to the door was a desk with a computer and phone equipment on it. I went for it and started to pull it out of its sockets and began throwing it.

By then Dawn had run back into the store and positioned herself between the store owner and me. She was being crushed as the two of us tried to get at each other. I could hear him telling his technician to call the police. It was a huge commotion.

Dawn eventually got me to leave the store where we waited quietly in our car for the police to arrive. She cried softly.

In no time, two squad cars arrived and began talking with the owner. I stayed in the car while Dawn got out to try and speak to the officers. She repeatedly said, "She has FTD." "She has dementia." "She has behavior Frontotemporal Dementia."

Eventually, one of the officers stood outside the car and began to talk with me through the window. I'm not sure of all the things he asked. I do know I kept trying to tell him that the store owner was a cheat and showed him documentation to support my claims.

During our conversation Dawn kept trying to help and provide answers. The cop became very firm with her and told her to remove herself. She flat out refused and said I have FTD and need her assistance. I'm sure Dawn was thinking, this is when she gets hand cuffed. But, after a stare-down the other police officer took her gently away yet was in within hearing distance.

I just sat in the car mulling over the events. I thought to myself "I've never been to jail before. It will be an interesting experience." "If I go to jail, I'm going to make this a very public event." "The store owner is a liar and laughed in my face." "My computer still does not work," etc. "I'm going to write a journal about this episode."

After some time, I heard Dawn thanking the officers and how they handled the situation very well. She sat down in the driver's seat and handed me our Police Services "Notice Prohibiting Entry Pursuant to the Trespass to Property Act" sheets. She looked at me seriously and said, "You know what you did was wrong. You can't just go around damaging others property." "Yup." I agreed BUT he didn't fix my computer!

The last two weeks, there has been a few significant incidences with me becoming extremely aggravated, verbally, and physically confronting. My apathy is apparent.

This latest incidence brings up a whole host of worries for Dawn. She got me off this time... but what about next time? If I am charged, due to my FTD, I will be tried in a Mental Health court. How can she physically restrain me when I'm so fired up? Who can help her in such situations? Will my periodical poor behavior and apathy continue to spiral down? Behavioral Supports Ontario is an initiative meant to enhance services for older adults with complex and "responsive" behaviors that stem from dementia, mental illness, or substance abuse.

My behavior has meaning. I was communicating my frustration about my computer not being fixed after having it for 10 days. I was lied to about sending me computer away when it was not. I was spoke down to. I was left with few alternatives to fix the computer.

Unfortunately, although the behavior has meaning it still does not make it appropriate or OK.

I worry about Dawn. It must be so terrible to see her partner of 13 years act in ways that are beyond her comprehension. For many care providers, the stress becomes too much, and they leave the relationship.

Dawn is putting together her plan in case a serious episode happens like this again. She is working on a strategy plan with her friends.

You may be asking yourself, why I would write about such a terrible thing. If I don't write about it, how will you know? How will you know our behaviors has meaning? Look past the stigma and learn why this happens. And that is why I choose to write about it.

Although orange is the new black, I'd rather not wear.

Where are the People with Dementia in Ontario?

Date: November 7th, 2015

By the numbers:

- "In Ontario alone more than 200,000 people are living with Alzheimer's disease in 2013."
- "1 in 10 Ontarians over 65 has Dementia."
- "Dementia is the #1 cause of disability in Canada."
- "Dementia costs us $50K annually per person."

When I was first diagnosed about three years ago with probable Frontotemporal Dementia, I did a great deal of research on dementia; in Ontario. I was shocked to discover so many people had this disease. Yet, when I tried to become part of an advocacy group, I discovered there are very few of them which comprise only people with dementia. Yes, there are many for the Care Partner, but not just for people with this disease.

On reflection, I realize this is when hubris took over me. I thought to myself how I was going to be the person with dementia who will unite the voices in Ontario. How hard could it be? There are over 200,000 of us!

Fast forward to today. The Ontario Dementia Strategy Plan has begun to host Round tables to gather initial data. There are spots reserved for people with dementia. (That's a great thing!). Yet, it has been a true struggle to find willing individuals who will sit up at this table and have their voice heard by the people who can help facilitate change.

I know, you are probably shaking your head and asking: "How can this be?" It's true – I assure you.

As a person living with dementia, I have done my best as an individual to push for representation. I have contacted government sources, media, academic people to try and convince them that we are the experts. And of course, I use our motto: Nothing about us, without us.

I'm afraid I have failed miserably to unit us.

I'm afraid the Ontario Dementia Advisory Group (ODAG) has failed.

I'm afraid local Alzheimer Societies have failed.

I'm afraid the Alzheimer Society of Ontario has failed.

It has been a true struggle to have people with dementia at these Round Tables. It has been a source of frustration for all involved.

In Ontario, there are some very active advocates with dementia. It is from this pool of people that the media contacts for interviews; researchers utilize their expertise; Alzheimer Societies use over and over for their different initiatives.

The reason for over-using this small pool of advocates is simple – other individuals with dementia have not stepped up to have their voice heard.

The question becomes: why? Why is there a lack of advocates with dementia? Why is it so hard to "find" someone who has dementia to participate in projects or opportunities to have their voice hear?

This is not just an Ontario challenge but rather an international issue.

For this to change, we must change the culture of what is involved in advocacy work. And we must continue to challenge stigma through education. In addition, the Care Partner must take a back seat and encourage their partner to speak for themselves.

The diagnosis of dementia is obviously a confidential one. Upon it, the doctor contacts the Alzheimer Society and informs them of this individual's diagnosis. This is when First Link kicks in. If the person living with dementia wants to involve the Alzheimer Society, the First Link program is introduced to them. Once again, all confidential. This person may join groups or other programs for socialization. There are many such things that are not under the Alzheimer Society umbrella but are private organizations.

How do we get to these individuals to encourage them to be advocates? Well, there are a couple of ideas to consider:

- At the point of first contact, by any organization, information is given to them regarding this topic and include examples to join.
- Match the newly diagnosed person up with another person with dementia. This is for support and education.

- All organizations should work with Care Partners in assisting them to encourage their partner with dementia to speak up and have their voice heard. It is all to often the Care Partner takes over the conversations and less and less is heard from the person with dementia.
- Provide funding to organizations like Ontario Dementia Advisory Group (ODAG) of which I am a Board Member. This funding will be used to recruit members through a media campaign. And, I know there are more, but I can't think of them.

We NEED people with dementia to be at the table and speaking up for themselves and for others who are unable. Help us. If you know of someone who has dementia, please encourage them to advocate.

And remember, advocacy takes on many different forms. It doesn't have to be speaking in front of an audience or being part of a Board of Directors. It could be the raising of one's hand in response to a question or taking part in a survey.

If Ontario wishes to have an Ontario Dementia Plan that truly has input from the experts, then we need to get the experts to the table.

I'm reminded of the great inaugural quote in 1961 from President John F. Kennedy: "Ask not what your country can do for you - ask what you can do for your country."

The time is NOW.

Lest we Forget

Date: Nov 11th 2015

I am humbled by this day of remembrance. Many of my ancestors fought to protect their country and their families.

Great Great Uncle - **Horace Wighton** 1866 – 1886 Private B Company Cameronians (Scottish Rifles) To be stationed in Jubbulpore, India

Buried: Western Cemetery, Maryhill, City of Dundee, Scotland

Great Uncle - **Horace Wighton** 1897 – 1918 WW1 - Regiment: South African Field Artillery, Unit Text: "A" Bty; Gunner. Buried:

Alexandria (Hadra) War Cemetery, Alexandria, Al Iskandariyah, Egypt, Plot A, 225

Great Cousin - **Horace Alexander Evans** 1924-1944 WWII

Flying Officer, Royal Canadian Air Force J26336 Division 625 (R.A.F.) Sqdn Buried: ST. HILARION COMMUNAL CEMETERY; Yvelines, France Grave 6

Grandpa - **Alexander Cromb Wighton** 1902 – 1967 WWII 1942 – 1945

Duty: Pipe Instructor. Train pipers who then were sent overseas to the European theatre.

Camp Ipperwash, Lambton county, Ontario, Canada

Dad – **William George Wighton** 1926

WWII 1943 – 1947

Army Reserve. Trained as a Gunner.

At age 17, Bill attempted to join the Navy. Although underage, he lied about being 18. He was turned down after his medical examine due to poor eyesight. He then went to the Army where they asked for proof, he was 18 years old. Caught, he was only able to enlist in the Army Reserve.

Grandpa Srg. **Fred Moran** 1894-1976

WWII 1915 – 1918 European Theatre

7th Canadian Mounted Rifles

Wounded: Sanctuary Wood, Belgium 1916

Great Uncle PTE. **Gordon Moran** 1897 - 1927

WWII Army 1916 - 1917

Mustard Gas poisoning in France; Died later from it.

Uncle **William Fredrick Moran** 1921 - 2014

WWII 1943-1945 European Theatre

Flying Officer with the Pathfinder Squadron RCAF

A Story of Two Brothers

A soldier's story can be is to be found in the service story of two brothers - Sgt. Fred Moran and Pte. Gordon Moran. They grew up on a farm in Sombra Township, but after their father died, their mother, a Moore

Township woman, moved them back to her childhood community of Courtright. Fred enlisted in 1915 and served with the 7th Canadian Mounted Rifles. He was injured in Ypres and was on administrative duty the rest of the war. When he returned home, he married, then became a sailor. He lived in Moore Township and died in 1971.

Gordon's enlistment was accomplished during the excitement of a military parade. The soldiers of Lambton County's own Lambton 149th staged a recruiting drive that saw them march from Sarnia down to Sombra and back to Sarnia. Caught up in the excitement of the moment, Gordon enlisted right there.

The Lambton 149th was a replacement battalion used to replace wounded or dead soldiers in other battalions. During his service overseas with the 2nd Pioneers, Gordon was a victim of an enemy mustard gas attack. The painful and destructive effects of the gas made it necessary for Gordon to return home to recover in 1917, but he died 10 years later in London from pulmonary tuberculosis. He is buried in St. John's Cemetery in Sombra.

YEAR FIVE

Shayla

Date: January 5th 2016

When Brianna started high school, she almost immediately began talking about her new friend, "Shayla." It wasn't long before Shayla became a permanent fixture in our house. We learned that things were tough in her home for her and her two siblings. In no time, we could usually expect her to be sitting at our dinner table and sometimes her brother would also join us.

When I reflect upon those early years of our relationship, I see a young girl struggling to simply survive in a tough world. As we came to know Shayla, beautiful, intelligent, hard-working, and determined person emerged. Like a diamond, after being found, she needed some polishing up. Our love towards her was the soft cloth used to help her shine.

Throughout the years, Shayla would live with us for a variety of lengths of time. She had her own bedroom which gave her a place to call her own. Her attempts to live out on her own didn't always work out. We always kept her bedroom for her for those occasions.

Our relationship wasn't just one way. She brought laughter to our home and the continual education of animals – which is Shayla's passion. She showed us that you must be determined to achieve your goals in the face of hardship. I think of the moment of her receiving her high school diploma. She had reached a personal milestone. It showed on her glowing face; We were so proud of her. And today, she is working towards being a Veterinary Technician.

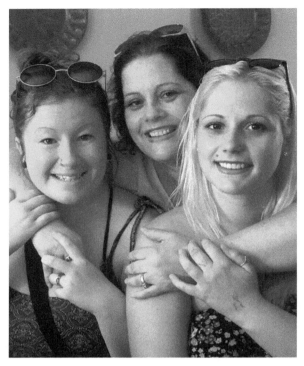

Shayla, Dawn and Brianna

As the years have ticked by, our relationship with Shayla has developed into one of parents and a daughter. Although Shayla is not my biological daughter, I do consider her to be my "adopted" daughter. And for that, I am honoured. It has been a joy to watch her develop into a loving, independent, confident, and caring individual. She has so much to offer the world. It's a better place since she came along.

They Still Make Me Laugh

Date: January 10th, 2016

The other day I was asked to share about myself. It didn't take long before I started to tell a group of others who I am. It went something like this:

My name is Mary Beth Wighton. I'm 49 years old. I was diagnosed with probable Frontotemporal dementia about three years ago. I have a wonderful partner, Dawn, of 14 years. Our daughter, Brianna, who is 21 lives with us in our beautiful new home in Southampton, Ontario. It is a small beautiful town on Lake Huron. We moved about a year ago from Kitchener. We just love it.

Yesterday, I received an email from an old friend asking how I was as she hadn't heard from me in a while. Part of my response to her was: "We bought a house here and moved in Dec. 22nd! We are thrilled with our home and even threw a New Year's party with some new friends! How fortunate I am."

These personal descriptions of myself have come to make me thing how much I have changed over 14 years in being with Dawn. When Dawn and I first met, I was in the prime of my career. I travelled a great deal around the world; made lots of money; had a cat named "Jack"; and was fiercely independent. I loved to read, watch good suspenseful movies and Taco Bell was my favorite fast food. I used to love to surprise Dawn with flowers – "just because" and learned that I had a creative side in making special cards for her.

When I met Dawn, I knew she was the one. The twinkle in her brown eyes told me so. And much to my delight and desire, she came as a package deal – Brianna was seven years old. I have the honour to be refereed to as "My second Mom" and "My MB."

Us three ladies have travelled through a lot of life together. We have had our ups and downs and all around! Through all of this we have striven to keep our core values: honesty, respect, and unconditional love. We have pushed each other to be the best we can be. Our faith has become stronger and we explore it together. We remind each other how blessed we are to have all that we do and to live in the great country of Canada.

If you would have asked me 14 years ago to describe myself, it would be so different from today. I would have told you about my career and things I owned and places I had been. I probably would have said how great I was at my job. I would have come across as confident and perhaps bore you with my success stories.

Today, all those things just don't matter anymore. During the same meeting where I was asked to share about myself, someone said how she realizes that after the meeting talking about dementia, that we then go back to our lives. How true this is.

Behind all my journals, my rants and raves about dementia; my outcry for change of people and government; my complaining about how I can't do the things I used to be able to do; squawking about how much my medication costs and the lack of a national dementia plan, there is much more to me.

I have an incredible life. I am much loved my many, by Dawn and Brianna. I live in Southampton because we choose to live Carpe Diem – to live for the day as we do not know what tomorrow may bring. In fact, we choose to do that each day. We make sure to get down to the Lake every day to look at the breath -taking ever changing scenery that God has given to us. When we have a party, we ask our friends to bring their kids and dogs because we love to have that type of noise in our home.

The other day, the three of us sat up to the table to have dinner. As we bowed our heads to give grace, Dawn broke out in song – Johnny Appleseed.

The three us all started to laugh. This was a song we used to sing many years ago with Brianna.

Behind my journals – My Girls still make me laugh.

The Table

Date: February 13th, 2016

When I think back to when I was a child, l has wonderful memories of our family sitting up to the kitchen table. It was a place where we started our day by eating breakfast at the table, and at the end of our day we regrouped and had dinner at the table.

Back in the day we didn't have cell phones to compete with for our attention and the TV was in the basement. It was a time where each one of us sat up to the table and shared about our day's events. It was a place where I learned about politics and the high price of gasoline. This was the place where we debated topics and after dinner was finished, we would wipe the table off and it became our place to play cards. It was also where I did my homework and wrote my essays. In other words, it was the center of our home.

Over 40 years later, the table still holds a revered place in our home. When Brianna was younger the house rules for when we ate at the table were no television and no cell phones at the table. Over the years, technology has fought for a place at our table. Brianna's friends would come up to the table with their cell phones. We politely discouraged them from using it.

Part of our routine was a blessing for our food, "cheers to the cook" and we would each share a part of our day. It was the few minutes where we would have undivided attention to connect.

It makes me smile to hear Brianna's friends reminisce about our table time. Today, they reflect on it and realize it was an important part in being plugged into Brianna's life. For those who did not have this within their own home, they have told me that they miss sitting up to the table with our family. It now brings back great memories for them.

Just over a year ago, we moved to Southampton and rented a small house. It was cute but didn't have room for a kitchen table. We decided we would make do for a while. For an entire year, we juggled our food on our small individual TV tables. As the days went by all three of us grew more discontented with this routine.

The situation changed just around Christmas when we moved into our new home. It had a dinning room area and would be a perfect place for our table. The problem now was that we had sold our table and didn't have one to put in this area. The search was on.

Dawn and I began to comb through stories and the internet. We knew we didn't want it to come out of a box and must be assembled. It was wood and Canadian made that where are guiding factors.

Yesterday we found it! In the Market in Southampton they sell Mennonite made furniture. The work is beautiful, well-made, and comfortable. At 5:00 pm yesterday it was delivered, and we had our first dinner on it. We oohed and awed and pointed out all the things we loved about the table and chairs.

The table was made by a local Mennonite family who has 10 children! It is a business where all contribute. It is a Harvest table made with 7 planks of pine with a dark walnut finish. The chairs are made of oak and are called ladder chairs. They are heavy and comfortable. It has a wonderful character to it as you can see the knots in the wood and other designs.

For the first time in over a year, My Girls and I sat up to our table. We fell right back into our routine of no TV or cell phones. We laughed and giggled and simply enjoyed each others company.

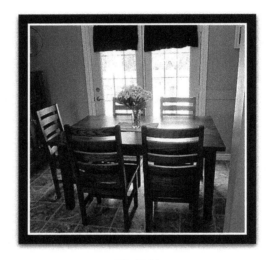

The Table

We look forward to having our family and friends over so they too can sit up to our table and connect with us.

So, if you are ever in our area, please stop by and pull up a chair to our table. We'd love to have you.

Making History

Date: March 24th, 2016

Advocacy work can be remarkably interesting. Sometimes, when you are in the 'thick of it' fighting for your cause, you may not even realize the impact you have until a third party points it out. This is what happened just a few weeks ago.

Nancy Rushford from Alzheimer Society Ontario approached the Ontario Dementia Advisory Group (ODAG) asking if we would like to participate in the First Link/Programs exchange conference that she was facilitating.

With Nancy, ODAG members discussed this wonderful opportunity and created a strategy on how two of our board members could use video conferencing technology to participate. Our other two board members would be in Toronto at the conference and would work directly with the participants.

The topic of the conference was partnering with people who have dementia. ODAG worked hard on its presentation with our own partners helping us create an awesome presentation – at least on paper. Now, the trick was to do it. What better way to learn about how we did then to hear it directly from the Keynote speaker? Here is what he wrote:

I had the privilege of witnessing history recently at an afternoon workshop given by the Ontario Dementia Advisory Group. This was the first-time people living with dementia were an integral part of a conference on dementia, in this case one sponsored by the Ontario Alzheimer's Association. After listening to ODAG's presentation and workshop facilitation it is clear there will be no turning back. The combination of their expertise and presence is too powerful and enlightening to ignore. I am confident that Friday, March 11th will be remembered as the start of a new period in the history of dementia support - a period in which the faulty assumptions about people with dementia are eventually overturned and the contributions of people with dementia are welcomed, expected and respected. How fortunate for all Canadians that ODAG has begun its pioneering work with such flair and confidence.

Was the presentation perfect? Of course not. But it is one heck of a great starting point for others to come!

Thank you to the many people and partners who support us, in particular:

- Centre for Education and Research on Aging and Health (CERAH)
- Murray Alzheimer Research and Education Program University of Waterloo (MAREP), and
- Mindset Centre for Living with Dementia.

What an exciting time in advocacy for people living with dementia. (Imagine the Rocky movie theme song starting to play…) Stay tuned… more great work to come.

Who Knew? Great Canadian Women

Date: April 12ᵗʰ 2016

I like to think of myself as a bit of a historian. As a young girl I could be found reading books on WWII Resistance groups and watching movies about war – and the people it impacted. It was really my insatiable curiosity and interest in people who, under duress and terrible circumstances, somehow rose above it and became everyday hero's. I always pondered if I would be a hero given the same circumstances.

Like many young Canadian historians, I didn't believe Canada had very "interesting" history as it was a young country and it lacked the many volumes of books about battles, royalty scandals and beheading, the Plague, etc. What my young mind didn't realize that was Canada is very rich it its history – it is just poorly documented. And what was captured in books, my young mind found boring.

The other day, I bought a magazine titled, "Canada's History." Hang on – don't stop reading yet! The magazine cover intrigued me – "20 Great Women" with numerous pictures of stoic looking women staring at me. In a split second, it hit me – I struggled to name 20 Canadian women who helped change history. How can that be?

The eyes of these women on the magazine cover burrowed into me. They challenged me to learn about each one of them. I flipped quickly through the magazine and was startled on how many names and faces I did not know. It got me thinking.

I have concluded that Canada had duped me. It intentionally did not provide the stories of these women to me as society, including education, supports gender disparity.

I can tell you that in 333 BC Alexander the Great was alive and kicking. How can I not know Nellie McClung's effort led to Manitoba being the first province to vote in 1916? I know that in the USA, Rosanne Parks, who was a black woman, refused to sit in the back of the bus (where she was supposed to due to her colour). Parks action ignited blacks in Montgomery Alabama to avoid using buses in protest of racist laws.

How can I not know that long before United States civil rights movements, Canadian Viola Desmond took a stand for racial equality in Halifax? In 1946 Desmond refused to sit in the theater section unofficially set aside for black patrons. She was dragged out, jailed for the night, and fined. Segregation was legally ended in 1954 Nova Scotia.

Agnes Macphail? Who knew she was the first women elected in the House of Commons and of the first to sit in Ontario's Legislative Assembly? And she initiated Ontario's first equal-pay legislation in 1951.

Adelaide Hoodless? Kenojuak Ashevak? Mary Two-Axe Early?

So, what the heck happened that I am not very well-educated in knowing great Canadian women who have had such an incredible impact on me as 1) a woman and 2) a Canadian?

Simple – I was not meant to. My education was designed that way. It was gender biased. No wonder I found Canadian history boring – I was only ever getting half the story!

As I ponder my latest realization of life, it hits me that a $7.99 magazine taught me more about many great Canadian women than I learned in my life (and that is with 6.5 years of higher education). Oh, by the way, my major was in history! It also makes me wonder what the current history curriculum looks like.

The last week has been terribly busy with me writing to parliament and national organizations pushing for the rights of people living with dementia. Would you be shocked if I told you that Canadian society continues to push for gender- biased solutions? You know the kind

– target the women folk, the "caregivers" of people. I have six brothers
and I know they are more than capable to also be a "caregiver."

When are we going to profoundly change Canadian history and
write, teach, and learn about great women figures in Canadian history?
And when are we going to stop implementing gender-biased national,
provincial, and local policies?

ODAG and the Canadian Senate

Date: May 23rd, 2016

After something of great significance has occurred in your life, it can
take a long time to mull over the impact it has on you – and potentially the world.

On April 11th of this year, on behalf of Ontario Dementia Advisory
Group (ODAG), I contacted the Clerk for the Standing Senate
Committee on Social Affairs, Science and Technology. There is a study
on dementia in Canadian Society. Part of the letter stated:

"Developing a cure must be the long-term goal of dementia policy
making. But supporting and empowering people with dementia and
their families should equally be an important policy goal. It is critical
that government uses the best available evidence to design appropriate
policies that affect people living with dementia.

The Standing Senate Committee on Social Affairs, Science and
Technology has been authorized to examine and report on the issue
of dementia in our society. Its website shows 14 Witnesses have or are
scheduled to provide testimony. The glaring gap in the witness list is
a person living with dementia representing the key stakeholder group.

The time is now to include people with dementia in contributing
directly to the examination of and reporting on the issue of dementia
in our society. Who better to learn from than people with dementia
who live the experience of dementia every day, who utilize programs
and services, and who are citizens within Canadian Society?"

Much to our delight, on April 22nd, I received the following response:

"This email is being sent to advise you that the committee would
like to invite you to participate in its public hearings on this study.

You are being asked to participate with a panel of 1 or 2 other organizations/individuals by making a brief statement (no more than 7 minutes) followed by a question and answer session with committee members. This session will last approximately 1.5 hrs."

I could feel my heart soar as our hope became a reality. ODAG would have the opportunity to speak for 747,000 Canadians who have dementia. We would be in front of Canada's policy makers to influence them on what people with dementia truly need.

Our next step was to request accommodation according to the Convention on the Rights of People with Disabilities (CRPD) to enable us to take part in our country's decision-making. The international community of people with dementia has recently started to use the strategy of demanding our legal rights described by the CRPD. Canada is listening and responded as I hoped it would.

The Senate made the following accommodations:

- I would participate via videoconferencing.
- Three Board Members of ODAG would appear in person in front of the Senate in Ottawa. Normally, only 1 or 2 from an organization can provide Evidence at one time. For ODAG, they accommodated the request to have 4 members present at one time.
- We had a total of 10 minutes as a group for an opening statement. Normally, it is 7 minutes.
- All 4 ODAG members could answer questions from the senators; not just 1 or 2 members.

ODAG already felt victorious with asking for and receiving accommodation as it applies to CRPD.

The entire ODAD team worked extremely hard in preparing for our presentation to the senate. This involved developing an Opening Statement. It was decided I would read it to the senate. In addition, we created a Brief to accompany our Witness statement. We came up with possible questions we would receive and strategized the best answers for them. Each senate member's profile was reviewed to best understand individual priorities and who were the key decision influencers.

It truly felt like all organizations and people who knew ODAG and worked with us was rallying behind. Offers of all kinds of support came pouring in. We had the assistance of Alzheimer Societies helping us in Ottawa.

The core team consisted of:

ODAG

- Myself.
- Bea Kraayenhof.
- Bill Heinbien, and
- Phyllis Fehr.

Strategic Partners:

- Laura Bowley, President, Mindset Center for Living with Dementia.
- Lisa Loiselle, Assistant Director, Murray Alzheimer Research & Education Program (MAREP).
- Nancy Rushford, Director, Alzheimer Society of Ontario.
- David Webster, Program Manager – Dementia Friendly Communities, Alzheimer Society of Ontario, and
- Dr. Elaine Wiersma, Associate Professor, Centre for Education and Research on Aging and Health.

Our final ODAG meeting prior to the senate was wonderful. We laughed, clapped, and congratulated ourselves for our achievements to date. Having the senate make accommodations for us according to the CRPD was an international victory for people with dementia.

Wednesday, May 18th, 2016 finally arrived. My ODAG counterparts had traveled to Ottawa and had arrived at the Victoria Building, just across from the Parliament of Canada. It houses the offices of parliamentarians, mostly members of the Canadian Senate.

The technical team set me up to videoconference the meeting. As I waited nervously from my desk in Southampton, I could see the senators filing into the meeting room. It was truly a special moment in my life.

With an introduction by the Chair, I began to read ODAG's Opening Statement. I spoke for about 8.5 minutes – just shy of the 10 minutes that had been granted to us. For the next two hours the senators asked their important questions from us to better understand what it is like with dementia in Canada. They looked to us for our opinions and warmly encouraged us by their dialog and tone of voice.

As each ODAG member spoke to their own experience, it became obvious how we were four people who lived very differently lives; had different experiences and support; and yet, came together as a team to implore the senators on the need for the Canadian government to create a national dementia strategy and to recognize the legal rights of those with dementia that are currently being denied.

When the Chair convened our meeting an hour longer than scheduled, ODAG knew we had made history. And what an indescribable feeling it is. I thank the many individuals who made this happen. It is something I will never forget.

I suppose you are wondering the impact we had on the senate. The Clerk says:

"I just wanted to touch base to once again thank you all for making extra efforts to participate in the Senate Social Affairs committee hearings yesterday. Even today the Senators were talking about how valuable they found your testimony to be."

Sue, Marie, and William Rudolph

Date: June 24th, 2016

Yesterday my dear friend, Sue, contacted me via Facebook. She had a link to a National Women's History Museum's photo of William Rudolph with the comment: "...reminds me of your speech in grade 5 or 6." Holy smokes! Sue remembered my grade 6 speech!

Today, my dear friend, Marie, added "I can totally see you picking Wilma Rudolph for a speech MB. Perfect fit!"

My two friends do not know how much their comments and connection to my past influences me.

I was brought back in time to my grade six class where I stood in front of my peers telling the story of William Rudolph. I remember the feeling of awe as I researched this first American woman to win three gold medals in track and field at a single Olympics. She was a member of the black community and regarded as a civil rights and women's rights pioneer.

What really impressed me was she recovered from polio, but it left her with a twisted leg and foot. Through treatment and adversity, she also overcame this physical challenge. She then began her sports career which would eventually earn her the Olympic gold medals and many awards and honours in years to come.

I have been struggling the past few weeks with my dementia symptoms. Apathy has been fighting for a spot in my life. It is important to remember that apathy is not depression. Apathy is a loss of motivation, marked by characteristics as diminished initiation, lack of interest and low social engagement.

This week I attended my first session of the Alzheimer's program "Minds in Motion." Beyond the obvious of being significantly younger than everyone, I would later realize I was struggling with "small-talk." Rather than making the effort to converse with the person sitting next to me, I preferred to just sit there and watch.

On reflection, I realize that I have been avoiding situations where small talk is involved. This includes talking on the telephone. I am fine during my ODAG meetings, as there are always topics to discuss and decisions to make. I'm quite happy being at home or out on my own without interaction of others.

In addition to apathy, my short- term memory also seems to be wavering. Last week, we had a dog trainer at our house to help me train our new dog, Sadie. I remember looking at Dawn, with tears in my eyes, as I couldn't remember the four steps necessary for her to sit, stay, look and "OK." Dawn kept encouraging me. It seems easy now.

In fact, I found Sadie who is a beautiful eight-month Husky, to be too much for me to manage. I became frustrated and annoyed with myself and her. Taking her for her much-needed walks, just seemed too much.

In addition to this, my good old boy, Shiloh, became gravely ill. Shiloh is a brown lab with a gray beard and is showing his 12 years. He is my partner in crime. Fortunately, he was able to pull-through and is on the road to recovery.

But we made the decision not to keep Sadie as it was just too much for me, Shiloh, and My Girls. A good friend of ours adopted her.

When Sue and Marie commented on Facebook about when I was a young girl, it brought me back to a place where I can remember. I can remember standing in front of the class; I can remember the feeling of being inspired by Wilma Rudolph; I can remember the feel and the smell of the library books written about her; I can remember.

I have a decision to make. I can buy into the "apathy is a sign of my dementia getting worse." Or, I can be like Wilma and fight through the pain, setbacks and continue to reach for the gold medals. I'm sure you know which decision I will pick.

Thank you, Sue, and Marie, for helping me remember!

The Big Event

Date: September 4th, 2016

The day started with a red cardinal looking straight at me. The house was quiet. I was the first one up in the house and was pouring myself a cup of coffee. I looked out our back window and saw the familiar black face staring at me. The red cardinal was so close to our home that it was almost inside. It stayed just long enough for me to get a glimpse at it. My angels were with me. I knew it was going to be a glorious day.

The day before, close friends started to arrive in Southampton to help Dawn get ready for the event. My brother David, good friends Phyllis and Tom, Shelly and her Mom had already arrived. We had been very busy preparing a crazy amount of food. Brianna and her friend Casey had taken over the living room. There were stickers, ribbon, brown paper bags everywhere. I was not allowed in the area.

The house began to awake. It was filled with laughter and instructions. The coffee pot kept brewing and brewing. The big day was finally here.

The cars began to leave the house for the destination where the shindig was being held. At 2:00 p.m. Shelly chauffeured me over to the party being held at one of the buildings at Dawn's work.

My 50th birthday party had begun!

Excitedly, I approached the building. It is one of those rounded steel buildings with a huge garage-like door. It had been transformed into an elegant party place. I just couldn't take it all in fast enough.

To the right side was tables and chairs all setup like it was a wedding. In the middle of each table was a bottle of wine with a picture of me on it and chocolate kisses strewn about. To the left of the room was a line of tables heaping with food. And then there was the carnival area: an air popcorn machine, candy floss maker and and a snow cone maker!! It was crazy.

Somehow, Dawn and her crew of helpers had transformed an ugly building into a beautiful area for celebration which included a photo area. A box of costume items including boas, hats, and crazy sunglasses was placed in the front of the room. This was the area where pictures were taken in front of a backdrop of a sign saying 50. Way too much fun!

And then a "candy bar" was setup so people could take home a "goody" bag. Yup, Dawn really knows me well!

The room quickly became a live with my family and friends and people who I had never even met! It was festive and fun. It was clear – the day was all about me celebrating my 50th birthday.

Since I was diagnosed with probable frontotemporal dementia in 2012, my life has become more enriched by people reaching out to me and making sure I know that I am loved and supported.

This is very much a contradiction to many who are diagnosed with dementia. Friends and family pull away from the individual because they don't know how to "deal" with it.

I am so grateful to say that I have not experienced that but quite the contrary. During our afternoon of celebration, I had moments where

I truly was overwhelmed by the love that electrified the room. I am so blessed to have so many people in my life who love me – regardless of dementia.

When I was first diagnosed, like so many others, I had been given a life expectancy of 2-10 years after diagnosis with an average of 6 years. Since there is no treatment to stop the progression, I am told that I will eventually advance to being completely dependent on care.

Somewhere in the back of my mind, I am aware of this, but I choose to ignore it. I work very hard to stay "in the moment "and to live each day the best I can. Yes: carpe diem. It was 23 BC when Roman poet Horace wrote this in his book of Odes. After all these years, it remains relevant and an important motto.

As I stood at the front of the party room listening to my family and friends sing happy birthday, I couldn't have been more in the moment. I truly was happy to celebrate 50 years of my life. And why shouldn't I be? I am living a wonderful life.

Dawn and I rarely talk about the time when I will become more dependent. Why bother? I have too much living to focus on. I have too many more birthday celebrations to participate in. Life is full of choices. I thank so many people for also choosing to celebrate with me. And, I thank Dawn and Brianna who are there every day of my life helping to live carpe diem.

Until my next birthday...

The Canadian Senate Listened!

Date: November 24th, 2016

There are few times in the average Canadians' life where the opportunity to influence how our nation thinks and responds about a particular topic occurs. I am one of the fortunate few to be able to capitalize on such an opportunity.

It was Wednesday May 16th, 2016 when I sat at my desk in Southampton and spoke to The Standing Senate Committee on Social Affairs, Science and Technology located in Ottawa. The Ontario Dementia Advisory Group (ODAG) had been invited to be a witness for its study on dementia in Canadian society. Our other three board members: Phyllis Fehr, Bill Heibein and Bea Kraayenhof were seated in the Senate room in Ottawa.

ODAG considered it a victory just to be in front of the Senate. We had worked hard to get there. We pushed for our rights as Canadian citizens with a disability to obtain concessions which allowed us to be better presenters. We had many people helping us to achieve this and many more cheering us on from the side lines. Who knows what you are capable of until you demand it from yourself and of others? I guess that's what called being an advocate.

In my speech I stated an especially important fact: "My story is like most other people living with dementia. It is our desire to live life fully and utilize our remaining skills that help us remain strong. We reject the notion of going home to die. The time between diagnosis and end-stage dementia can be many years. In the meantime, we have the ability to live life well."

After ODAG finished its presentation, we congratulated ourselves, partners, and supporters. We had done our work, now it was time for the Senate to do theirs.

For just over five months, the Senate has been reviewing the many hours of expert testimony given about dementia. It is interesting in that there were many well-known people who had spoken great words of wisdom and presented spirit-crushing facts about its impact. We were the unknowns – desperate to make an impact with our own voices – the ones with true experience of living with dementia. The question now is, did the Senate hear us?

The answer came on November 15th, 2016 in an extensive report release titled "Dementia in Canada: A National Strategy for Dementia-Friendly Communities. It stated, "A fully-funded National Dementia Strategy is urgently needed to support caregivers, research efforts and Canadians living with dementia." Wonderful!

Within the report, there is a chapter called "The Patient Perspective." My answer to the question on if we were effective was answered: "Of all the expert testimony offered throughout this study, none was more compelling than that which was given by members of the Ontario Dementia Advisory Group..."

We had done it! Four average Canadians living with dementia had managed to communicate our expert witness perspective. The Senate had not only listened but truly embraced our words and did their best to make sure all of Canada also heard us.

I felt like a superstar as congratulations poured in. I'm so proud of ODAG and our very important partners. This moment has negated the many times when I have shouted out in rage and despair. It is the moment that I will keep near and dear to my heart and pull out when I need to remind myself that I have made a difference.

My love of Canada just deepened as I have participated in democracy to fight for my rights.

How about you? If you want change don't be afraid to stand-up and shout from the mountain topics. If we do not – then how can we expect things to change?

4th C.M.R. Battalion Operation Order No. 17

Date: November 10th, 2016

Grandpa Moran (Sgt. Fred Moran) used to say he had two belly buttons. The scar of a shot wound through his stomach, became his "second belly button."

My Mom would tell the story of him being a soldier in the Great War. He was 21 years old and was part of the 7th C.M.R. Battalion, which initially was a horse regiment prior to being shipped from Canada to France. It was October 21st, 1915 when he joined the battalion in the field. This was a far cry from this sailors' job of ship captain on the Great Lake Huron.

The War Diary of the 4th C.M.R. Battalion, Operation Order 17 tells us of what Grandma Moran and his comrades were instructed to wear and to bring to battle.

On the morning of June 2nd, 1916, the German bombardment – on the front lines – intensified. In the fiercest bombardment yet experienced by Canadian troops, whole sections of trench were obliterated, and the defending garrisons annihilated. Four large mines detonated under Mount Sorrel. Human bodies and even the trees of Sanctuary Wood were hurled into the air by the explosions. As men were literally blown from their positions, the 3rd Division fought desperately until overwhelmed by enemy infantry.

That day, the 4th Canadian Mounted Rifles had casualties for all but 76 of their original 702 men. Grandpa Moran was one of those wounded that day. A German bullet found its way to his stomach causing him to fall on the battle ground. He would later tell the story of lying there for hours until nighttime came. Using the protection of darkness, he would be rescued and brought back to safety.

The battle at Hill 62 and Sanctuary Wood lasted a total of 5 months and the result of careful planning and strategy earned Canadians their pride and bravery in the Great War. But as always, there was a heavy price to pay for their success. 8430 Canadians died fighting in this battle.

Grandma Moran was one of the few who survived. He would forever carry the physical and emotional battle scars of not just Sanctuary Woods but the Battle of the Somme, Vimy Ridge and Passchendaele.

In January 1919, Grandpa would return from the depths of hell to somehow embrace his life and freedom. He would obtain his Marine Master's certificate, marry, and become a father to five children.

I sometimes think of Grandpa, laying wounded in the mud. I wonder what he thought about as bullets whizzed past his head, shrapnel flew overhead, and he listened to the cries of wounded soldiers from both sides. I wonder how many times in his life his mind would bring him back to the horrors of war. I wonder.

I wonder when this world is going to stop fighting.

As I always have, I am so thankful for being Canadian and living in this great country. I was reminded of how lucky I am this week, when the web site for how to move to Canada was flooded with requests from the United States to the point where the server stopped working.

My heart thanks Grandpa Moran and the many, many, many soldiers who have fought and fight to preserve the way I live. I will always remember.

Poverty and Dementia

Date: December 10ᵗʰ, 2016

I have a heavy heart tonight. I'm restless. I have felt like this for the last few days.

It started when I was doing research on "Adequate standard of living and social protection" for Canadians with disabilities. My search brought me to: Monitoring poverty and social exclusion 2016 Click for report. It stated: In 2014/15, there were 13.5 million people in poverty in the UK, 21% of the population. It then went on, "Once account is taken of the higher costs faced by those who are disabled, half of people living in poverty are either themselves disabled or are living with a disabled person in their household."

These numbers shocked me. I suppose I have my head down in the sand and think of poverty like this is in the third world countries – not the UK.

As you may already know, older women are at higher risk. Simply put, they live longer; many had the sole career of taking care of their family – and therefore do not have pensions or they are smaller than that of males; and they are usually the prime care giver and rely on family and friends when they are in crisis.

At an intellectual level, I know these facts. National papers use them in their headlines just this past April 2016, Ontario's poverty gap for single adults on welfare has skyrocketed by 200 per cent over past 20 years. And this is without reference to people with disabilities - dementia.

And what about the electricity rates? Yes, Ontario pays among the highest in North America. The latest poverty type – "energy poverty."

Being a person with dementia, numbers can be quite challenging for me. It is challenging to understand them and the implications of them. It is, therefore, easier to just focus on one person with dementia living in poverty and what it means for them. So, let me tell you a story.

"Jean" was just diagnosed with dementia. She lives on her own. A friend of mine, "Luke" who also has dementia, reached out to Jean with the intent to provide support. During their chat, Luke began to ask basic questions about her welfare. He quickly realized Jean was in serious trouble. Jean was confused about benefits she is entitled to. She had little food in her fridge; was not taking medication because of its costs; wasn't sure how she was going to pay her rent, etc.

This I understand.

Luke immediately began to help Jean with signing-up for the benefits she was entitled to including the delivery of Meals on Wheels. It took him hours over the phone. Without Luke, I'm not sure what would have happened to Jean.

When I was younger, I went to Haiti on a "Poverty Experience." The stench of poverty will never leave me. The children with big eyes, and protruding bellies due to lack of food is forever ingrained in me. And it was worse with people of disabilities. The slums in Port-Prince are some of the worse in the world. It is a world of its own – people just trying to survive each day.

And then there is Ontario's Poverty Reduction Strategy 2014 – 2019. It comments on a "multifaceted, complex problem." hmm.

I keep thinking about Luke and Jean. Does this have to be such a complex problem to tackle? Jean is a person in our community. Yes, even yours. But where are the Luke's? Where is our humanity? Our concern for the frail in our communities?

Just saying.

Congratulations ODAG – It Has Been Quite a Year!

Date: December 14th, 2016

The Ontario Dementia Advisory Group (ODAG) has enjoyed one heck of a great year.

It is only two years ago that we formed in the fall of 2014 with the purpose of influencing policies, practices, and people to ensure that we, people living with dementia, are included in every decision that affects our lives.

I am so incredibly pleased to share with you that ODAG has truly helped in breaking down stigma and educating our politicians, medical and research communities, retirement and long-term care and Canadian citizens. We have done this through:

- Speeches
- Presentations
- Videos
- Blogs
- Meetings with government representatives
- Position papers, etc.

In addition to this, we also have demonstrated how much more inclusive it can be for people with dementia when we use technology – in particular, Zoom. This provides a proven two-way communication method allowing for people to participate in our important work, regardless of where they live.

How did we accomplish all of this? Hard work, incredible ODAG supporters, and through constant improvement, pushing the envelope and sheer determination.

We have achieved so many successes that there are too many to list. To choose just one - it must be ODAGs Witness presentation to the Canadian Senate on the study of dementia in Canadian senate. Reading its report, our impact on this Standing Senate Committee on Social Affairs, Science and Technology is quite obvious: "Of all the expert testimony offered throughout this study, none was more compelling than that which was given by members of the Ontario Dementia Advisory Group, Mary Beth Wighton, Phyllis Fehr, Bill Heibein and Bea Kraayenhof."

I'd like to thank ODAG's Board Members for their dedication and perseverance: Phyllis Fehr, Bill Heibein, Bea Kraayenhof, Tammy Bellamy, and Carole Johanneson. This could not be done without you!

The ODAG partners are true partners and we are so fortunate to have them: Lisa Loiselle (MAREP), Dr. Elaine Wiersma (Centre for Education and Research on Aging & Health) Laura Bowley (Mindset Centre for Living with Dementia), Nancy Rushford (Alzheimer Society of Ontario), Lauren Rettinger (Alzheimer Society of Ontario), Kirsten Broders (Centre for Education and Research on Aging & Health) and Emily Fraschetti (MAREP).

Dad – Happy 90th Birthday!

Date: December [30th], 2016

Some of my earliest memories is of my Dad and I doing things together. When I was about four years old, my Dad and brothers built a garage. Instead of telling me to stay clear and get out of the way, I had a job – I was the nail straightener. With my hammer I had the responsibility to hammer out any crooked nails so they could be re-used. My Dad grew up in the depression, so we never threw out things. He patiently showed me how to do it, and away I went. To me this was much more fun than playing with dolls!

I'm guessing I was about grade 3 when Dad gave me my first pocketknife. I made good use of it with the apples in Germain Park. I also tried my knack at whittling. I'm not sure if my Mom knew about my new tool.

And in grade four, Dad had me cutting our grass with a push lawn mower. I can remember feeling how great it was that he trusted me to do this. And that same year I was helping by trimming our hedge.

On reflection of my relationship with my Dad, it is one of him encouraging me to be the best I can. It has been a consistent message for my 50 years of living. By having expectations of me and pushing me to do things by myself, he has played such a positive influential role in helping to develop the very core characteristics of my being.

I think perhaps the most important advice I have received comes from my Dad. I was 18 years old and trying to figure out what to do with my life and what university I should attend. In his wisdom he stated to me that it doesn't matter what I did for my career, but to ensure that it was something that I can always depend on to support myself and my family. He shared how important it is to have a reliable job that provided financial security and not to rely on my spouses' job. What would happen if my spouse became sick and died? I have always remembered that conversation and it has guided me in many choices I have made over the years.

Dad was born in 1926 in Sarnia, Ontario. The tough economic times of that day greatly influenced the shaping of him as a person.

His parents were part of the working poor. When he was 16 years old, he quite school and began to work full-time at Imperial Oil. He would work there for 43 years before early retirement due to medical issues. Dad also grew up helping to support his Mom and two younger brothers. His father was away due to WW2. Dad had to grow up fast.

December 25th is an important date not just because of the birth of Christ, but also because it is my Dad's birthday. I think that if you are a Christmas Baby, you must be extra special. Because that is what my Dad is.

Just a few days ago, Dad turned 90 years old. My family threw a great birthday party for him. In addition to his family, my aunts, uncles, and cousins attended the event. It truly reflects how Dad has played a role in many peoples lives other than my own. He is so loved for who he is – a gentle, kind man.

Even today, Dad still encourages me to be the best advocate I can be. He tears up with pride. I have always, always known that he will wrap his arms around me with unconditional love.

I am so thankful to him for so many things - being an amazing example of a husband, Dad, Grandpa, Father-in-law, friend, and neighbor. We are so fortunate to have this man for 90 years. In fact, he is still teaching us by his actions.

Happy 90th birthday, Dad!

YEAR SIX

Coordinated Care in Ontario's Health System

Date: January 29th, 2017

What would make it easier for people with dementia, their care partners and care providers to navigate available services and supports?

One of the biggest hurdles for people living in Ontario with dementia, partners and care providers is the ability to navigate easily and successfully available and supports. To understand what is needed to make it easier, we need to understand the current status quo.

Currently, there are gaps in dementia care including lack of support and training for care partners, poor care transitions and inconsistent access to community-based services. A result of this inconsistent quality of care is preventable episodes of emergency department visits and hospitalizations.

After years of seeing many doctors and specialists, I was finally given a diagnosis of probable frontotemporal dementia. With the diagnosis, I was told to get my affairs in order and my driver's license was revoked on the spot. To help my partner and I through this I was given a pamphlet about FTD and the instructions to contact the Alzheimer's Society as they are the experts.

Like many other people with dementia, I was contacted by CCAC to determine how they could help us. Much to my dismay, it too only had one pamphlet on FTD; the day programs were for people over 55 – I was only 45 and was told that I could not go to it; all other programs were geared towards people with Alzheimer's – which I don't have.

Not finding the support I needed, my partner and I began to comb the internet for information and support services. I mean there must be other people with FTD! The medical and support system failed us. And it is still failing us.

Each person, at the time of diagnosis, should expect the same type of support that any person with a disease would receive. For instance, a person with a diagnosis of cancer will automatically receive support based on the "Disease Pathway Management Program" that develops and maintains pathways that depict current evidence-based best practice for the diagnosis of all major cancers. Each person with a cancer diagnosis can expect a team of different health care professionals – doctors, nurses, pharmacists, dietitians, social workers and other. They are there to treat the cancer and to help the patient and family.

Why do I not receive the same types of supports that a person with any other disease receives?

So, the question is what would make it easier to navigate available services and supports. A great deal of research can be found on this topic. There are several proposed solutions. The one strategy that really stands out is the creation of a position, somewhat like a case-manager, called "Dementia Consultants." These positions are created in collaboration between local governments, health-care organizations, and health-care insurers.

The Dementia Consultant provides advice and support across sectors to different target populations and in the different phases of the disease with the aim to improve the quality of life of the person with dementia.

We know that there are many different supports available for both the person with dementia and their care partner. There is a need for more care continuity. The Dementia Consultant can coordinate the match between demand and provision across phases and sectors and ease the transitions between different care providers.

An example of a Dementia Team that could be coordinated includes:

- Family Doctor
- Nurse
- Patient Advocate
- Pharmacist
- Dietician
- Occupational Therapist
- Musical Therapist
- Physiotherapist

- Social Worker

- Dementia
  Specialist Doctor

- Financial Adviser

- Spiritual Care Worker

- Art Therapist

Web-based Navigation

In addition to a Dementia Consultant Role there are other possible solutions to help with the navigation of services and supports. Instead of having a person help in navigation, a single point of navigation for dementia can be web-based.

This site can direct users to web based community support and activities, peer-support groups, including web-based community support and activities, online information and advisory services, and an online dementia road map. For me and my partner, the internet has really been an important source of support and information. It could be even better, to have some type of dedicated web site.

Rise Up!

Date: February 26th, 2017

I can remember when I was young being called a Feminist. I wasn't too sure what the word meant, but it was said in a context that made me think it was a "dirty" word. So, of course I denied it. No, I wasn't a Feminist!

And then when I was older and knew what the word meant; it still had a "dirty" word feeling to it. Once again, I denied I was a Feminist – but, I did believe in equality of the sexes! Somewhere along the way, the definition of feminism for me was not a word of empowerment but rather a radical, risky way to describe oneself. And then for women who did say there were feminist a nasty group of people usually called them a "bunch of dykes."

It was/is complicated as a young woman to find the inner courage to stand up for herself and act in a manner that is respectful and self-loving.

Women in management and leadership roles, including myself, have had to deal with off-coloured comments about our management styles. If a man acted in the same manner, there wouldn't be such comments.

I now say I am a Feminist – and I say it proudly. The definition of a feminist has not changed since I was a young girl. It is I who has changed, matured, and have grown confident in my own beliefs. It still is "A feminist is a person who believes that men and women are equal (though not necessarily the same), and should be entitled to equal rights, equal treatment, and equal opportunity."

Over the last few months, I have watched in fascination and awe, the world coming together and rise up! On January 21, 2017, over three million women boarded buses and took to the streets in the United States. Across the world, women followed in an incredible movement with the message: women matter.

"We the people" has taken back its meaning and refers to all people regardless of sex, race, religion, and sexual orientation. We are once again at a moment in history where the people have had enough and are rising up. The Women's Marches around the world is one of power and unison. It is a reminder for all of us that we can make a difference – we just need to keep adding more people to the cause.

It is also the time to teach our young ones, regardless of sex, that feminism is not a "dirty word" but one of power and pride. Teach them young.

The time to stand up for our human rights has never been greater. Feminism is just one component of it. Reader – Rise Up!

She's One in a Million

Date: March 12th, 2017

Last weekend was a special date for me. My Partner, Dawn, and I celebrated 15 years of being together. And we did just that – celebrated! We hopped in the car and took a leisurely drive down the lake road. Our destination was a quaint town with the best sushi restaurant in the area.

In true form, Dawn and I talked and laughed as we reminisced our years of being together. We rarely have the radio on as we seem to always have so much to say to each other. The radio is just a distraction.

n arrival to our destination town, we immediately drove down to the lake. We both are in awe of the beauty of nature. And today was no exception. There were ice burgs just off the shore. A true Canadian scene of splendor. We then headed to the towns main strip to browse through a few stores.

We finally entered the quaint restaurant that is supposed to have the best sushi. We were the only people in it which was simply perfect. Neither one of us is too adventurous when it comes to sushi, so we stuck to what we already knew we would enjoy. And of course, we had to order some take-out for Brianna.

Dawn has changed in many ways since we first met. And in other ways she hasn't. I always enjoy watching how she interacts with people. She oohs and ahhhed to the server about the food and the restaurant. While down at the beach, she got into a conversation with some folks who were also out walking. And she is always on the look out for someone who needs a helping hand or a kind word. It's what I love about her.

The last month has been a difficult one for us. We have lost a dear friend to cancer. Our hearts are heavy. But we look from signs from heaven to help cheer us up – and that's exactly what the red cardinals do as they sit on our bird feeders.

It seems that there is always a constant reminder of how precious our relationship is and life itself. Our motto of carpe diem has served us well. We do our best to stay in the moment and enjoy each other and the simple things of life. It can be quite easy to get lost in the "what if" or "when this happens..." of my dementia stages. Our conversations about what is important to us and to remain true to ourselves are incredibly important.

I know that it has not been easy on Dawn to have a partner who has a terminal illness. It must be frightening to think of what is to come. And therefore, it is so important for us to stay in the moment. Many partners of people who have frontotemporal dementia leave them. It is too difficult for them and so they leave the relationship.

I know as I'm changing, I am less sympathetic and more self absorbed. My short-term forgetfulness has taken another notch up. I sometimes see Dawn's frustration, but then she bites her tongue. It must be difficult to watch my abilities change.

This only has seemed to make Dawn stronger. She is my partner and does anything and everything to help me live the best way I can. I would expect nothing less of her because that's the kindness she has in her heart. And I love her for that.

It is hard to believe 15 years has already gone by. Time truly does fly.

In today's world of chaos, I am so fortunate to have My Dawnie Girl. She truly is one in a million.

Being the Chair of ODAG

Date: April 3rd, 2017

It seems like a long time ago when the founding members of the Ontario Dementia Advisory Group (ODAG) discussed the creation of a group for people with dementia run by people with living with dementia.

In October 2014, five people living with dementia and members of key Ontario organizations came together to discuss the possibilities of an Ontario dementia advocacy group. The group consisted of:

Nancy Rushford	Program Director at the Alzheimer Society of Niagara
* Maisie Jackson	Person living with dementia
* Bea Kraavenhof	Person living with dementia
Gina Bendo	Alzheimer Society of Niagara
Delia Sinclair	Alzheimer Society of Ontario, Public Policy and Advocacy
Phil Caffery	Alzheimer Society of Ontario, Public Policy and Programs
Lisa Loiselle	MAREP, University of Waterloo

* Brenda Hounam	Person living with dementia
* Mary Beth Wighton	Person living with dementia
* Bill Heibein	Person living with dementia
Elaine Wiersma	CERAH, Lakehead University

* Founding members living with dementia.

Over the course of time, except for me, all founding members living with dementia have left the group for a variety of reasons. And all individual partners have also departed except for Nancy Rushford (no longer with the Alzheimer Society), Lisa Loiselle, and Elaine Wiersma.

In a period of 2.5 years, this is a lot of movement for any group. And that's not a good thing. Relationship building takes time and effort, and this is even more so for people living with dementia. It also takes a hit on moving our agenda forward as members leave with knowledge and experience that our new members do not yet possess. Think of it like the ebb and flow of water.

Further to that, our organization partners also have their own agenda and budgets that may affect ODAG. Staff positions become redundant, etc. And plans that we had in using certain resources once to available us, are removed. Challenging to say the least!

When ODAG decided to be an advisory group, the Ontario Dementia Strategy plan was in its infancy. The Board Members thought it made great sense to make supporting this strategy as our top priority. We pushed our way into several the various groups and demanded we had representation at the table. We also adopted the famous movement disability motto: "Nothing about us, without us." To that, we fought to represent ourselves and not have organizations, advocacy groups or our care partners do it for us. We became a force to be reckoned with. As time went by, ODAG members proved their value and insight into the strategy plan. And with this came numerous invitations to participate in projects, groups, speaking engagements and panel conversations.

We were becoming noticed not just at the provincial level - the international world was taking notice.

One area that ODAG has always struggled in is the recruitment of new members at large and new board members. In early conversations one partners made the following comment regarding obtaining information on advocacy groups in Ontario: "...the list of the local advisory groups that have formed—unfortunately, we haven't collected that information. At this point, we're not sure about who's doing what. Hopefully, the provincial group can connect with the local groups as we hear that they are forming?"

We are still struggling to connect with individual in these groups. Why? It can be for several reasons:

- Lack of confidence in the person with dementia (PWD)
- Not wanting to make a commitment
- Unaware of ODAD
- Afraid of using the technology of Zoom
- Not interested in advocacy work.

"Nothing About Us without Us"
Huge Ontario Budget Win

Date: May 1st, 2017

For many people living with dementia, our partners and supporters, the Ontario budget 2017 was a great success for us. When ODAG formed in the Fall of 2014, the original Board Members decided to create a group that would focus on creating a loud single voice of those living in Ontario who are living with dementia; and to do this through applying pressure on the government to create and fund a provincial strategy. I'm so pleased to say that we have won a huge win with allocation of money for this important plan. There are many faces and names who have come before me and have walked with me during this struggle to gain "power for the people." I hope this wonderful news reaches them and they can finally say, "At last." Congratulations to all of us! And now... the next stage – implementation!

Below is ODAG's release to the media:

For immediate release

Ontario Dementia Advisory Group commends the Ontario Government for investing in a dementia strategy

Toronto, ON - April 28, 2017 - The Ontario Dementia Advisory Group (ODAG) is thrilled with the Government of Ontario's commitment of $100 million over three years to launch a province-wide dementia strategy and congratulates Premier Kathleen Wynne, Minister Charles Sousa and Minister Eric Hoskins for making dementia a priority.

"Better dementia care is no longer an option - it's a necessity, which is why a dementia strategy in Ontario is crucial," says Mary Beth Wighton, Chair of the Ontario Dementia Advisory Group.

The Advisory Group is also pleased with the Government's $20 million pre-budget investment in resources and supports for care partners, who are most often family members.

"There is still much work ahead of us to make sure the needs of people living with dementia are recognized and met by the provincial health-care system. The Government's commitments are a critical first step to getting us there, so that every person with dementia lives with the highest quality of life," says Wighton.

The Ontario Dementia Advisory Group was formed in 2014 and comprises of individuals from all walks of life who are living with dementia and who work together to influence policies and practices and ensure their voices are heard.

For media inquiries:

Mary Beth Wighton, Chair, Ontario Dementia Advisory Group

Why Do You Not Believe Me?

Date: July 2nd, 2015

When I say I have dementia, there is usually a stigmatized response: "Gee you don't look sick." "You are too young to have dementia." "I'm not good at math either." "Everyone gets forgetful."

What I find surprising is that some of these stigmatized responses come from people who know me, have direct contact with me and are recipients of my advocacy work. It is as if they don't believe I have a disease that has no cure and ultimately will die from. One such person said that I "...can walk and talk so I'm fine."

What else do I need to do for all people to believe me?

Perhaps the better question is why do I feel the need to convince them? And why am I disappointed, hurt and sometimes angry with them that they don't?

Rest assured I have received a diagnosis of probable Frontemporal dementia. I have been through the gamete in seeing doctors, tests, and been under high scrutiny. My brain has been picked and prodded at. I'm so sick of it, that I have told Dawn I'm done with doctors and don't want to see and more. I will do the basic requirements necessary for me to retain my personal insurance. That most likely means a yearly visit to the world-renowned brain hospital Baycrest to see the Head, Division of Neurology.

I'm reminded of the apostle "Doubting Thomas" who refused to believe that the resurrected Jesus had appeared to the other apostles until he could see and feel the wounds of Jesus.

Skeptic, why do you not believe I have dementia?

I am unable to show you my diseased neurons that are not firing on all cylinders. I am not alone in this as most people having dementia experience this stigma. I am fortunate in that I have an early diagnosis. This has enabled me to have the time and ability to learn about my diagnosis and prepare accordingly.

Dementia does not mean I am old and always forgetful.

Skeptic, I:

- am a person
- have a diagnosis of dementia
- have great long-term memory
- struggle with short-term memory
- struggle with making decisions
- struggle with math
- struggle with understanding humour
- struggle with understanding complex movies
- struggle with word finding
- am not as compassionate to others as I once was;
- take a great deal of medication that makes me tired (not lazy), and
- I am loved by many.

Reader take the time to understand dementia. It doesn't take long. Educate yourself. I would hate to think that you too are a skeptic.

Great Great Uncle Horace: His Sad Tale

Date: November 9th, 2017

It was a few years ago while I was doing family research, I came across the tragic story of my great great Uncle Horace C. Wighton. I was told we had a Wighton curse on the name Horace. Anyone with this name and was a Wighton has died a horrific death. This was certainly true for my great great uncle.

He was born in 1866 in Kinnoull, Perth, Scotland and were one of six children. The 1881 Scottish census shows him working as an agricultural labourer at the age of 14. The next time I was able to find him was in the Glasgow Herald newspaper – on three different occasions. Below is the story of a young soldier who was so frightened by the thought of war that he made the decision not to go.

Glasgow Herald - Saturday 23 January 1886

"MYSTERIOUS OCCURRENCE AT MARYHILL BARRACKS

MYSTERIOUS OCCURRENCE AT MARY HILL BARRACKS. A mysterious occurrence took place at Mary Hill Barracks yesterday morning. The men of B Company of the Cameronians (Scottish-Rifles) discovered on rising that Private Horace C Wighton, one of their number, was absent. The blankets on his bed were found to be smeared with blood, while a blood-stained razor and a small pool of blood were on the floor near the bed. Wightons' clothes were all in the room with the exception of his drawers and socks. The police were at once informed of the matter, and an examination was made. Footprints and occasional blood spots were found on the snow in leading in the direction of the canteen. Here the wall was scaled which led into the ground at the Garrison Hospital. The marks were traced across the ground and then outside the iron railing at the west side of the hospital. From this point the footmarks were traced along the drill ground at intervals of about 4ft. to the side of the river Kelvin, where a halt seems to have been made, as both footprints were close together. Slightly the mark of the left foot was seen, the probable conclusion being that a leap had been made into the water. Inspector Beddie of the civil police assisted by the military, searched the river all day until darkness set in, but no further traces were discovered. Wighton was only about 20 years of age. He a was a native of Perthshire, and only returned to the barracks after a 21 days furlough. He was of a quiet and retiring disposition. He was one of the draft which is about to proceed to India from the Scottish Rifles and made it no secret of being averse to going abroad but nothing unusual in his behaviour was observed on Thursday eight."

"Glasgow Herald - Saturday 20 March 1886

THE DISAPPEARANCE OF A SOLDIER FROM THE MARYHILLS BARRACKS – A body, which is believed to be that of a soldier Horace Wighton, who disappeared from Maryhill Barracks on 22 January, was found in the river Kelvin yesterday afternoon. The throat was cut, and the body was much decomposed. On the morning of Wighton's disappearance from the barracks the blankets of his bed were found to be smeared with blood, while a blood-stained razor was found on the floor near the blood. Footprints and blood spots were found on the snow leading in the direction of the canteen; and outside the barracks the marks were traced to the bank of the Kelvin. Search was made by the military and police authorities, but nothing further regarding the missing man was discovered. Wighton was a private in B Company of the Scottish Rifles, about 20 years of age, and a native of Perthshire. He was to have been on a draft of the regiment which recently proceeded to India, and was understood to be averse to going abroad."

"Glasgow Herald - Saturday 27 March 1886

MARY HILL-MILITARY FUNERAL-The remains of Horace Wighton, a private in the Scottish Rifles, were interred yesterday afternoon in the Western Cemetery, Maryhill, with the usual military honours. Wighton, it will be remembered, disappeared from Maryhill Barracks on Friday 22 of January, and his body was recovered in the river Kelvin on Friday last. The W.S. Shanks, of Maryhill Church, conducted the service, and a firing party of 14 fired three volleys over the grave."

John Wighton, brother of my great great Uncle Horace had to come and identify the body of his younger brother. The death certificate stated, "Supposed suicide by drowning."

What I find surprising is that he received a full military honours funeral. I am grateful he did.

How many more people have done the same thing – yet, the story was not told in a newspaper? How many more people will die in war? One more name…one more cause…one more war.

As always on Remembrance Day, I ask myself, "How many more must die?" How many more great great Uncle Horace's' will be taken from their families. I wonder.

Tribute to Shiloh

Date: December 16th, 2017

It happened five weeks ago. I knew it was coming.
You knew too but just kept humming.
We met 13 years ago. You sat so good.
The rest of our dogs never would.

We picked you because we knew you were best.
No other dog could pass the test.

Your big floppy paws made us laugh and then holler.

Shiloh, Shiloh how I miss your brown eyes and your green collar.

You quickly grew into a handsome furman.
That all could depend on, even Batman.

I whispered my secrets in your big floppy ears.
They always felt like cashmere.

I loved when you romped and made angels in snow.
Your warm brown eyes always continuing to glow.

The kittens and cats, the other dogs too,

Always took over your bed, no bother to you.

Shiloh, Shiloh how I miss your brown eyes and your green collar.

Your hips were so bad, so typical of Labs.
They stopped you from running but swimming was fab.

Your bed lies beside us. It still smells of you.
I can't bear to remove it as it reminds me of you.

Your grey beard grew fuller as I was diagnosed sick.
Your mission on earth began to click.

Your snoring reminded me to laugh when I was down.
How could I possibly give you a frown?

I know you're in heaven where all good dogs go.
Sitting by St. Peter, paws at his toes.

Shiloh, Shiloh how I miss your brown eyes and your green collar.

Government of Canada Hosts National Dementia Conference: Inspiring and Informing a National Dementia Strategy

Date: May 28th, 2018

When I was diagnosed six years ago, I never thought it would be possible that Canadians would gather in Ottawa and work together to discuss and begin definition of the first Canadian strategy. It's happened!

Last week a group of about 175 people converged on Ottawa in an invitation-only National Dementia Conference fulfilling a key component of the *National Strategy for Alzheimer's Disease and Other Dementias Act*. Approximately 25 people living with dementia attended as did many of our care partners. The conference brought together a broad range of stakeholder groups and partners from across the country and internationally to help inform a national dementia strategy.

In addition to this the Honourable Ginette Petitpas Taylor, Minister of Health, announced the establishment of a Ministerial Advisory Board to advise her on matters related to the health of persons living with dementia. The Board, which will be co-chaired by Dr. William E. Reichman, President and Chief Executive Officer of Baycrest and the Centre for Aging + Brain Health Innovation, and Pauline Tardif, Chief Executive Officer of the Alzheimer Society of Canada, will represent people living with dementia, their caregivers, researchers, advocacy groups, and health care professionals.

Of the 15 people on the Ministerial Advisory Board, two people who have dementia are part of this team. Jim Mann, from British Columbia and myself have the incredible honour to sit at the table as equals with the other members to advise the Minister.

My heart is bursting with pride for the MANY people who have helped to make this day possible. Some of the original ODAG Board members including: Brenda Hounam, Beatrice Krayenhof, Bill Heibein and Maisie Jackson set the stage for what we can accomplish when we work together on a common goal.

New Board Members joined the team, including Phyllis Fehr, Tammy Bellamy, Carole Johannesson, and Keith Barrett who spent many, many hours helping to define the first Canadian group of people living with dementia fighting for ourselves. We challenged status quo on every step of the way and fought our way to present to the Canadian Senate acting in our own capacity as Witnesses.

In addition to the Board Member team, we have many ODAG members who support each other from rural Ontario to the urban areas including Toronto.

We could not have done it without a very special group of partners including: Lisa Loiselle from Murray Alzheimer Research and Education Program (MAREP), Dr. Elaine Wiersma, Director of the Centre for Education and Research on Aging & Health and Associate Professor in the Department of Health Sciences; Gina Bendo from Alzheimer Society of Niagara Region; Nancy Rushford from Alzheimer

Society of Ontario, and Laura Bowley, Director at *Mindset Centre* for Living with *Dementia*. Please forgive me if I have missed your name.

And of course, the backbone to our work is the many un-named and unrecognized partners who help us be all that we can be. A special thanks goes to my Dawnie Girl.

In Canada, we have now moved into a new era of advocacy for people living with dementia, where our focus is less provincial/territorial and more national in scope.

It was one of my most memorable moments in my life to attend this conference with Dawn and meet others from across Canada. Some I have know for years but had never met. Their hugs told their many stories.

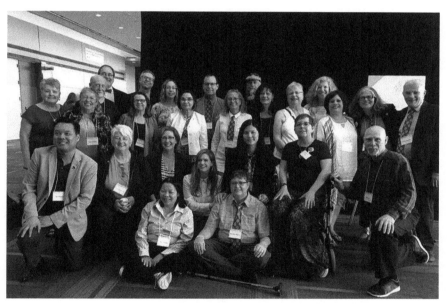

May 15TH 2018 Ottawa, Canada. National Dementia Conference

I'm truly humbled by this moment and can only express my sincere thank you for the many unnamed advocate heroes.

A new dawn has risen; I look forward to facing it with you, hand in hand, step-in-step with one voice. To guide us, Maya Angelou words of encouragement: "*You may not control all the events that happen to you, but you can decide not to be reduced by them.*"

A Boy, A Dog, and a Bottle of Root beer

Date: July 29th, 2018

I guess I have a lot to update you on. Writing my journals does not come so easily anymore. I have great topics and stories to write about but transferring those thoughts to paper has become a challenge. That's life.

It's already been eights months since we brought a puppy into our world. Since the passing of big brown lab, Shiloh, there was a gap in our hearts and our home. After a lengthy search by Dawn, we found Bailey – an apricot coloured cockapoo (Cocker Spaniel and Poodle mix). Bailey requires a whole book of journals to describe all his shenanigans! We love him even if he does bark too much.

In addition to Bailey, a young boy named Hayden also entered our lives. He has been spending a few days with us each week. We are helping to provide stability to this young man's life as his own home environment is unpredictable. Dawn and I have happily taken on the role of a surrogate grandparent. Hayden has a set of amazing grandparents who take care of him the rest of the time. Hayden is an incredibly smart, colourful, loving little boy. He is a delight.

As you most likely know, the mix of a boy and a puppy provides great entertainment. It also provides much needed medicine for The Fog. The thing about kids and puppies is they are non-judgemental and just want to love you. You don't have to remember the right words or what day it is.

Yesterday Hayden, Bailey and I had a wonderful day of laughing, playing make-believe and digging in the flower-garden. It started off in the dog-park across the street. Hayden's amazing imagination had us tip-toing through the jungle; fighting with the lions; digging a hole for the bag full of gold and protecting the king. He also dug a hole for our new flowers; helped put some food scrapes into our neighbour's compost barrel and fed Bailey his supper. Bailey simply just ran along with us wagging his tail – until he jumped into the neighbour's fish-pond – but that too is another journal!

Yesterday was such a carefree day for me. I didn't feel my mind was still in The Fog. My cognitive gears seemed to be working at optimum level. I didn't feel any pressure. I was pulled into Hayden's world of imagination and loved it. We ran across the park with our "swords" yelling at the lions and tigers.

And this three-year old is already learning about our birds: cardinals, finches, and back-headed chickadees. He filled up the bird feeder with sunflower seeds and watched with delight as the birds came to have a snack.

You may have noticed that I didn't' mention anything about electronics or T.V. Well, Hayden prefers to use his imagination instead of pushing buttons. He prefers to be outside to feel the sun on his back than being inside the air-conditioned house. And he prefers to run with Bailey than sit.

It makes me wonder. I wonder if the true medicine to The Fog is simply a young boy and a dog. Suppose we develop communities that encouraged relationships with our young and cognitively impaired? Many video's have captured this wonderful relationship. Wouldn't this be so much better than the "orange pill?"

Oh, and a bottle of Root beer? Well, that the best drink to have after a busy and long day of playing hard. Cheers!

A Boy, A Dog, and a Guitar

Date: August 28th, 2018

The other day, late in the afternoon, I tried to remember if I had a nap. I then realized I really didn't remember much about my morning at all. Unlike Alzheimer's disease, Frontotemporal dementia does not affect the memory in its early stages. I have noticed a change in my ability to remember, so I'm guessing things are getting worse.

But what I did remember was my afternoon with our young friend three-year old Hayden. I have become very fond of this young boy. He certainly brings out my inner child – my capacity to experience wonder, joy, innocence and playfulness. He can so easily bring me into his world of make-believe.

We headed across the street to the park, our puppy Bailey straining at his dog leach and Hayden dragging a long slender stick which he dubbed a guitar. What is so great about this long stick is that it also can easily transform into a dangerous sharp sword for a knight in shinning armour, a horse for a cowboy, or a weapon to kill the slithering snake in the jungle.

Bailey can easily transform into a fire-breathing dragon or an excited fan cheering on The Guitar Man. And me, well this is when my inner child appears. I can become anything that Hayden needs from me.

As we roared and giggled and ran to save the princess, the world of dementia disappeared.

Hayden's love for guitars comes from watching his "Grampy" play in a successful local band. Hayden is the band's number one fan and even has the honour of placing his real guitar up on a stand beside the band's instruments. As the Band belts out their tunes, our young musician can be seen nodding his head to the rhythm and stamping his foot.

My favourite song that Grampy sings is "You are my Sunshine." This is the song that Grampy and Hayden sing together. It is sung with such tenderness and love. As the two sings together, the crowd and band simply disappear. The only thing in my line of vision is Grampy and Hayden. I feel honoured to witness such a beautiful moment:

Although my memory seems to be sliding, the feeling that is left with me when I have spent time with Hayden and Bailey remains. It is one of peacefulness and satisfaction. And the sight of him playing his guitar... well, how can I ever forget that?

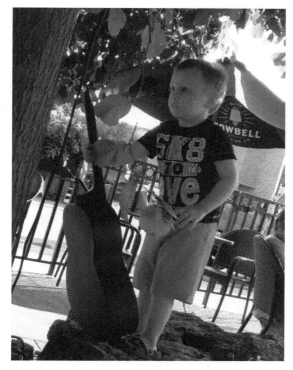

A Boy and his guitar

The Apple of My Eye

Date: Sept 10ᵗʰ, 2018

My daughter Brianna is 'the apple of my eye.' A long time ago, the pupil of the eye was called the 'apple.' It was thought that the pupil was much like an apple. When you look at someone, their reflection appears in your pupil. So, if someone is the 'apple of your eye' she is someone you look at a lot and enjoy seeing.

Brianna was seven years old when I entered her life. In six days, she will be turning 24 years old. My Mom used to say: "the older you get the quicker time flies." How true it is!

I am so thankful for having the honour of being one of two Mom's in her life. I have watched her grow – overcome obstacles – and succeed in reaching goals. And as of late, I have really seen her mature into an adult.

For years, Brianna has thought of becoming a Personal Support Worker (PSW) but only kept it as a career possibility while exploring the culinary world. This pass September, that changed. She was accepted into the PSW program and has begun the necessary schooling to obtain its certificate. I'm so very proud.

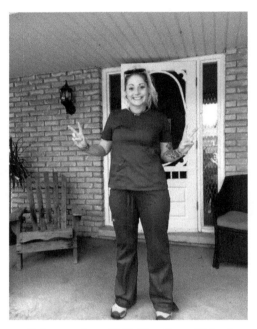

Brianna - Sept. 2018 First Day of School

One of the first topics to be covered in the course is dementia. Now, I sometimes think she looks at me a bit differently. I wonder if the words she has heard about my disease has triggered some emotions that we possibly haven't spoken about. Because I 'don't look like I have dementia' I suppose you can be lulled into the false sense of security that I'm alright. But I'm not.

Last week I was contacted about participating in a project that involves young carers and the technology for enabling them to get support through a digital network. This is a bit of a stretch for me and its not in my usual roundhouse of types of projects I work on. And that's when I realized that it really is Brianna that is the expert and would be an awesome team member. So, we have signed up together to help in this especially important and much needed project. I truly look forward to accomplishing this with the team, but mostly with Brianna. I'm sure we will learn much from each other during its design.

I know that the life of a PSW is a hard one. The work may be physically and emotionally demanding. And, it certainly doesn't make the Sunshine List in compensation. What I hope for Brianna is that she will have a rewarding career and know she is making truly a difference in peoples lives.

And of course, should the day come that I need a PSW, well I hope the apple-of-my-eye will hear my call. She is the one who knows my idiosyncrasies – the type of beer I like and the yummy candy and baking I crave. She knows the type of movies and books I enjoy. But most important, she loves me – and I her.

Carpe diem, Brianna.

Where is Our Moral Compass?

Date: Dec. 16, 2018

I did not sleep soundly last night. The energy of this world is changing, and my mind and body feel it. I try not to follow too much news. It makes me shake my head in disbelief.

I can remember being in high school around 1984 and working on a history essay. The Cold War was in its last few years with the USSR and the United States involved in a costly arms race. My essay was about the use of intercontinental ballistic missiles. The likelihood of such a missile being used to attack seemed real.

One of the most dramatic changing moments to end this Cold War was on June 12th, 1987, when President Reagan challenged President Gorbachev to tear down the Berlin Wall. In a speech next to the wall, Reagan stated: General Secretary Gorbachev, if you seek peace, if you seek prosperity for the Soviet Union, Central and South-East Europe, if you seek liberalization, come here to this gate; Mr. Gorbachev, open this gate. Mr. Gorbachev tear down this wall! And we know from history – he did just that.

Fast forward to today. Instead of having a U.S. President encouraging to tear down walls – we now have a President issuing Executive Order 13767, titled Border Security, and Immigration Enforcement Improvements, by President Trump on January 25, 2017. The order directs a wall to be built along the Mexico-United States border. Initially, he tweets (a new communication method for some Presidents) the Mexicans will pay for it and now he looks to the Military to build it.

And Reader, who knows what side of the Wall Debate you stand on?

How ironic that just over 70 years ago, when the world was recovering from the global horrors of WWII, the international community vowed never again to allow atrocities like those happen again. Under the brilliant chairmanship of Eleanor Roosevelt – United States President Franklin Roosevelt's widow, the newly formed United Nations' Human Rights Commission, created the Universal Declaration of Human Rights. The historical Declaration had over 50 Member States participating in its drafting of 30 statements.

The entire text of the UDHR was composed in less than two years. At a time when the world was divided into Eastern and Western blocks, finding a common ground on what should produce the essence of the document proved to remain an immense task.

So… here we go again; violations of basic human rights: Escalation of conflict of international political powers; war; borders; hate crimes; mass human migration; camps; famine; sex-trafficking; and religious extremism. The list goes on.

And Canada – once known for our Peace Keeping missions – has its own blemishes. As of 2013, more than 50% of the world's publicly listed exploration and mining companies were headquartered in Canada. Many of those companies have been accused of being irresponsible, engaging in conduct they could never get away with in Canada, exploiting weak or corrupt governments and legal systems in foreign countries that turn a blind eye to their operations.

What has happened to us? Why are we repeating the same things we did over 70 years ago prior to the development of the Human Rights

Declaration? Where is our individual and national moral compass guiding us to "do unto others as we would have others do unto you"?

We can change this world (again). But we must work to do it. We must stand up against the many different evils that is leading us and get back to the basics – human basics.

I can't think of a better way to end this than from the words of Eleanor Roosevelt: Where, after all, do universal human rights begin? In small places, close to home - so close and so small that they cannot be seen on any maps of the world. Yet they are the world of the individual person; the neighborhood he lives in; the school or college he attends; the factory, farm, or office where he works. Such are the places where every man, woman, and child seek equal justice, equal opportunity, equal dignity without discrimination. Unless these rights have meaning there, they have little meaning anywhere. Without concerted citizen action to uphold them close to home, we shall look in vain for progress in the larger world.

Introducing Bailey

Date: Dec. 18, 2018

It was about 14 months ago, when we had to put down our 13-year-old lab, Shiloh. It hit the family and our friends hard. He was one of those dogs that everyone loved. I believe I have been mourning him for all this time.

The gap in our hearts needed to be filled and this meant getting another dog. It was a tough topic to discuss as it was still soon after Shiloh died. But Dawn set about looking to find our next furry friend. She did a great deal of research and made numerous calls. It was narrowed down to a mixed breed – Cockapoo (Cocker Spaniel & Poodle). We liked the lapdog size; hypo-allergenic; intelligent; wavy hair; and low to medium energy level. Once we decided on the breed, the next step was to find 'the one.' The search was on.

Last year about this time, the family was in Toronto for me to receive an award. It was a very big deal and we were excited to go to the gala and celebrate. And of course, during all this, Dawn found 'the one.'

After the gala, and late into the evening, Dawn negotiated the terms, talked to the breeder, and agreed to a 5:00 a.m. time to meet 'the one.' The seller lived in Toronto and had to leave early for work, so the meeting had to be done before that.

With coffee in hand, Dawn and I drove to the apartment where we meet the puppy. We were excited and chattered about all the things we love about puppies. When the owner opened his door, we saw a little fur ball run behind his legs and began barking. Oh, he was cute!

He shared the story of "Bruno" being an apartment puppy and this was his first time owning a dog. He said he didn't realize the work that was involved in owning one and he was just not doing a good job. Hands were shaking and away we went with "Bruno."

We then went back to the hotel to pick up Brianna and Shayla. Much to their delight, we surprised them with our new family member. Our next stop was to show off our new member to Aunt Carol who lives in Toronto. Bruno received approval with lots of hugs and kisses. The car ride back to Southampton was filled with laughter and a few tears. Immediately, we knew Bruno was mine as he attached himself to me immediately.

When we arrived, the first thing we did was change Bruno's name to Bailey. He seemed much more like a warm and fuzzy dog than a brute. And then we introduced him to the beach. He was no longer a city dog but now was a beach dog. Life is good.

Our family has always loved animals. We encourage our friends to bring their dogs over as we our "pet friendly." And for me, having animals is incredibly important for my welfare. It is obvious the effect they have on me. Bailey truly calms me down; gives me a sense of responsibility and makes me laugh. I have struggled with remembering the training signals, so he could be trained to do many things, but we haven't bothered.

Since my diagnosis, I have always told the importance of animals on people living with dementia. They have an instinct that seems to help us feel better. Now, that's true medicine. And this is even the case for the mechanical animals that many residences now have adopted – like "Ageless Innovations Golden Pup Interactive Robot Toy Dog."

There are so many cats and dogs that need adopting. Many, who are a few years old, would make wonderful pets. But never forget it is a huge commitment and not to take lightly.

As I am writing this, Bailey has been busy trying to bury his bone under some blankets. He has kept me amused. What a great way to start my day. Thank you "Mr. Wigglebum" for helping me keep healthy and happy.